Kilian Eyerich

**Interleukin-17 is a key cytokine in first-line defence of the skin**

Kilian Eyerich

# Interleukin-17 is a key cytokine in first-line defence of the skin

Südwestdeutscher Verlag für Hochschulschriften

**Impressum/Imprint (nur für Deutschland/ only for Germany)**
Bibliografische Information der Deutschen Nationalbibliothek: Die Deutsche Nationalbibliothek verzeichnet diese Publikation in der Deutschen Nationalbibliografie; detaillierte bibliografische Daten sind im Internet über http://dnb.d-nb.de abrufbar.

Alle in diesem Buch genannten Marken und Produktnamen unterliegen warenzeichen-, marken- oder patentrechtlichem Schutz bzw. sind Warenzeichen oder eingetragene Warenzeichen der jeweiligen Inhaber. Die Wiedergabe von Marken, Produktnamen, Gebrauchsnamen, Handelsnamen, Warenbezeichnungen u.s.w. in diesem Werk berechtigt auch ohne besondere Kennzeichnung nicht zu der Annahme, dass solche Namen im Sinne der Warenzeichen- und Markenschutzgesetzgebung als frei zu betrachten wären und daher von jedermann benutzt werden dürften.

Verlag: Südwestdeutscher Verlag für Hochschulschriften Aktiengesellschaft & Co. KG
Dudweiler Landstr. 99, 66123 Saarbrücken, Deutschland
Telefon +49 681 37 20 271-1, Telefax +49 681 37 20 271-0
Email: info@svh-verlag.de
Zugl.: München, TU, Diss., 2010

Herstellung in Deutschland:
Schaltungsdienst Lange o.H.G., Berlin
Books on Demand GmbH, Norderstedt
Reha GmbH, Saarbrücken
Amazon Distribution GmbH, Leipzig
**ISBN: 978-3-8381-1756-0**

**Imprint (only for USA, GB)**
Bibliographic information published by the Deutsche Nationalbibliothek: The Deutsche Nationalbibliothek lists this publication in the Deutsche Nationalbibliografie; detailed bibliographic data are available in the Internet at http://dnb.d-nb.de.

Any brand names and product names mentioned in this book are subject to trademark, brand or patent protection and are trademarks or registered trademarks of their respective holders. The use of brand names, product names, common names, trade names, product descriptions etc. even without a particular marking in this works is in no way to be construed to mean that such names may be regarded as unrestricted in respect of trademark and brand protection legislation and could thus be used by anyone.

Publisher: Südwestdeutscher Verlag für Hochschulschriften Aktiengesellschaft & Co. KG
Dudweiler Landstr. 99, 66123 Saarbrücken, Germany
Phone +49 681 37 20 271-1, Fax +49 681 37 20 271-0
Email: info@svh-verlag.de

Printed in the U.S.A.
Printed in the U.K. by (see last page)
**ISBN: 978-3-8381-1756-0**

Copyright © 2010 by the author and Südwestdeutscher Verlag für Hochschulschriften Aktiengesellschaft & Co. KG and licensors
All rights reserved. Saarbrücken 2010

# Table of content

| Chapter | Title | Page |
|---|---|---|
| | Table of content | 1 |
| | Published data from the manuscript | 4 |
| | Used abbreviations | 6 |
| 1. | **Introduction** | 7 |
| 1.1 | Differentiation of CD4+ T cells | 7 |
| 1.2 | Non CD4+ T cell sources of IL-17 in the skin | 9 |
| 1.3 | Th17 cells and known effects of IL-17 in the skin | 11 |
| 1.4 | The skin as a first-line defence organ of the organism | 12 |
| 1.5 | Chronic mucocutaneous candidiasis | 15 |
| 1.6 | Atopy and atopic eczema | 21 |
| 2. | **Aim of the study** | 24 |
| 3. | **Materials and methods** | 25 |
| 3.1 | Patients | 25 |
| 3.2 | Materials | 27 |
| | Biologic material | 27 |
| | Cell culture material | 27 |
| | Chemicals | 28 |
| | Cytokines and antibodies | 29 |
| | ELISA systems | 30 |
| | Machines | 31 |
| | Used media | 31 |
| 3.3 | Methods | 33 |
| | Isolation of peripheral blood mononuclear cells | 33 |
| | Isolation and characterisation of skin-derived T cells | 35 |
| | Isolation and generation of antigen-presenting cells (APC) | 37 |
| | Stimulation and co-culture experiments | 37 |
| | *In vivo* experiment | 38 |
| | Flow cytometry analysis | 38 |
| | Enzyme-linked immunosorbent assay (ELISA) | 39 |
| | RNA isolation and Real time PCR | 39 |
| | Statistical analysis | 40 |
| 4. | **Results** | 41 |
| 4.1 | CMC patients suffer from an impaired secretion of IL-17 and IL-22 | 41 |

|  |  |  |
|---|---|---|
|  | CMC patients exhibit reduced total number of IL-17 producing T cells but normal amounts of CCR6+/CCR4+ T cells | 45 |
|  | PBMC of CMC patients are able to secrete Th17-differentiating and -maintaining cytokines | 47 |
| 4.2 | IL-17 is involved in a pro-inflammatory *circulus vitiosus* in atopic eczema | 48 |
|  | IL-17 producing T lymphocytes are infiltrating the skin during an APT reaction: newly characterized Th2/IL-17 subset | 48 |
|  | A subpopulation of Der p 1 specific T cells has the capacity to produce IL-17 | 54 |
|  | Stimulation with cognate antigen induces IL-4 and/or IFN-$\gamma$ release, but no or very low amounts of IL-17 | 54 |
|  | Th17 associated cytokines IL-1$\beta$, IL-6 and IL-23 do not increase IL-17 secretion in allergen-specific stimulated effector T cell clones | 56 |
|  | Staphylococcal enterotoxin B induces high secretion of IL-17 by Der p 1-specific T cells | 56 |
|  | IL-17 strongly induces HBD-2 *in vitro*, but this effect is diminished in AE | 58 |
|  | SEB strongly upregulates HBD-2 mRNA and protein release in Der p-induced atopic eczema *in vivo* | 60 |
| **5.** | **Discussion** | **61** |
| 5.1 | CMC patients suffer from an impaired Th17 immune response | 61 |
|  | The role of Th17 cells in *Candida* infections | 63 |
|  | CMC patients suffer from an impaired Th17 immune response | 63 |
|  | Th17-differentiating cytokines are not diminished in CMC patients | 63 |
|  | Mechanisms of candidicidal activity of IL-17 | 64 |
| 5.2 | The IL-17 mediated host defence is partially impaired in AE patients | 66 |
|  | IL-17 producing T cell populations infiltrating AE lesions | 66 |
|  | Secretion of IL-17 in T cells is tightly regulated | 66 |
|  | The role of the local microenvironment for the induction of HBD-2 in keratinocytes | 67 |
|  | A new concept on the pathogenesis of atopic eczema | 68 |
| **6.** | **Summary** | **70** |

| 7. | **References** | 71 |
| 8. | **Acknowledgement** | 85 |

**Published data from the manuscript**

**Original articles:**

**Eyerich K**\*, Pennino D\*, Scarponi C, Foerster S, Nasorri F, Behrendt H, Ring J, Traidl-Hoffmann C, Albanesi C, Cavani A. Interleukin 17 in atopic eczema: linking allergen-specific adaptive and microbial-triggered innate immune response.
J Allergy Clin Immunol. 2009; 123: 59-66.   (Impact Factor 2008: 9,7)

**Eyerich K**\*, Foerster S\*, Rombold S, Seidl HP, Behrendt H, Hofmann H, Ring J, Traidl-Hoffmann C. Patients with chronic mucocutaneous candidiasis exhibit reduced production of Th17 associated cytokines IL-17 and IL-22.
J Invest Dermatol. 2008; 128: 2640-5.   (Impact Factor 2008: 5,3)

\* Both authors contributed equally to this work.

**Review articles:**

**Eyerich K**, Foerster S, Hiller J, Behrendt H, Traidl-Hoffmann C. Chronic mucocutaneous candidiasis from bench to bedside.
Eur J Dermatol. Submitted.   (Impact Factor 2008: 2,0)

Foerster S, **Eyerich K**, Behrendt H, Ring J, Traidl-Hoffmann C. Rolle von Keratinozyten in der Pathophysiologie des Ekzems.
Allergo J. Issue 2. 2008.

A part of the experiments shown in this work was performed in the Istituto Dermopatico Dell'Immacolata (IDI-IRCCS) in Rome.

## Used abbreviations

| | |
|---|---|
| % | Percent |
| Ab | Antibody |
| AE | Atopic eczema |
| APC | Antigen-presenting cell(s) |
| APE | aqueous pollen extract |
| APT | Atopie Patch Test |
| Aqua dest. | Destilled water |
| Bet. | Betula alba |
| BFA | Brefeldin A |
| °C | Degree Celsius |
| cAMP | Cyclic Adenosine-monophosphate |
| CCR | Chemokine receptor |
| CD | Cluster of differentiation |
| CLA | Cutaneous lymphocyte associated antigen |
| cpm | Counts per minute |
| DC | Dendritic cell(s) |
| DNA | Desoxy-ribonukleic acid |
| EBV | Ebstein-Barr virus |
| ELISA | Enzyme linked immunosorbent assay |
| FACS | Fluorescence activated cell sorter |
| Fig | Figure |
| FcεRI | high affinity IgE receptor |
| Foxp3 | Forkhead box p3 |
| g | Gravitation |
| GM-CSF | Granulocyte-Macrophage colony stimulating factor |
| h | Hour(s) |
| ICAM-1 | Intercellular adhesion molecule 1 |
| IDEC | Inflammatory dendritic epidermal cell(s) |
| IFN-γ | Interferon-γ |
| IgE | Immunoglobulin E |
| IL | Interleukin |
| LC | Langerhans cell |

| | |
|---|---|
| MACS | Magnetic antibody column separation |
| MHC | Major histocompatibility complex |
| min | Minute(s) |
| ml | Milliliter |
| mM | Millimolar |
| MTP | Mikrotiterplate |
| mRNA | messenger Ribo-Nucleic-Acid |
| nm | Nanometre |
| NF-κB | Nuclear factor κB |
| PBMC | Peripheral blood mononuclear cell(s) |
| pDC | Plasmacytoid dendritic cell(s) |
| PHA | Phytohemagglutinin (= Lectin) |
| PI | Proliferation index |
| PPT | Pollen Patch Test |
| Phl. | Phleum pratense L. |
| PP | Poly-Propylen |
| µg | Mikrogram |
| µl | Mikrolitre |
| µm | Mikrometre |
| R | Receptor |
| rpm | Rounds per minute |
| REM | Scanning electron microscop |
| sec | Second(s) |
| Tc1 | Cytotoxic type 1 T cell(s) |
| Tc2 | Cytotoxic type 2 T cell(s) |
| TCR | T cell receptor |
| Th1 | T helper type 1 cell |
| Th2 | T helper type 2 cell |
| TNF-α | Tumor necrosis factor α |
| T-reg | T regulatory cell(s) |
| TRAIL | TNF related apoptosis inducing ligand |
| TSLP | Thymus stroma lymphopoeitin |
| U | Unit(s) |
| UV | Ultra-violet light |

# 1 Introduction

T lymphocytes are central mediators of adaptive immunity. Increasing knowledge regarding morphology, secretional profile and chemokine receptor repertoire of T cells reveals that distinct T cell subpopulations fulfil specialised tasks. Among these T cell subpopulations, much attention has been focused on interleukin-17 (IL-17) producing Th17 cells in the last years. IL-17, also produced by other T cell subsets and NKT cells, seems present especially in inflammatory and autoimmune diseases of epithelial tissue in the human organism. Accordingly, many *in vitro* studies demonstrate important tissue-instructing functions for IL-17.

In this context, the presented thesis illuminates that IL-17 is a central mediator for protection of the human organism against microbials at barrier-defining organs. This essential capacity is illustrated in two human diseases that are characterized by chronic and selective infections of the skin – the orphan syndrome chronic mucocutaneous candidiasis (CMC) and the common inflammatory skin disease atopic eczema (AE). This manuscript illustrates that CMC patients suffer from a generally diminished IL-17 response. In contrast, in AE IL-17 can be triggered efficiently by microbial-derived stimuli, but the local microenvironment in the skin partially inhibits an effective IL-17 response. In both cases, the absent or ineffective IL-17 signal results in a failed instruction of an innate immune response by epithelial cells, which can explain a selective inability to clear skin infections.

Taken together, this work describes that defence against extracellular microorganisms at barrier-organs such as the skin is critically mediated by IL-17, thus indicating that within T helper cell subsets the Th17 cells may be classified as "tissue-signaling leukocytes".

## 1.1 Differentiation of CD4+ T cells

CD4+ T cells orchestrate the adaptive immunity by mediating CD8+ cytotoxicity and phagocytosis by macrophages, by enhancing antibody production of B cells and by recruiting other leukocytes such as neutrophil, eosinophil and basophil granulocytes to sites of infection. They do so by the production of an arsenal of cytokines and chemokines – amongst these IL-17 (Figure 1). So far, at least eight distinct CD4+ T cell subsets are known. Th1 cells produce IFN-$\gamma$, induce apoptosis and are proinflammatory, Th2 cells are characterised by production of IL-4 and induce an eosinophil and mast cell immune response[i,ii]. Nothing is known about the function of Th9 cells that differentiate out of Th2 cells and are characterised by secretion of IL-9[iii]. Th17 cells co-produce IL-17 and IL-22, and they accumulate in several autoimmune diseases[iv]. Recently, a T cell population characterised by the production of IL-22, but not of IFN-γ, IL-4 nor IL-17 was discovered. These so-called Th22 cells are associated with inflammatory skin diseases[v,vi,vii]. Finally, T cellular immune responses are limited by a further independent entity of so-called regulatory T cells. These comprise naturally occurring CD4+CD25+ T regulatory cells (nTreg), inducible Treg cells (iTreg) and CD4+CD25- Tr1 (producing TGF-β) and Th3 cells (producing IL-10). While naturally occurring Tregs suppress effector functions of other T cells via contact-dependent mechanisms, iTreg, Tr1 and Th3 cells exert their suppressive activity via secreted cytokines[viii].

All known CD4+ T cell populations with the exception of Th9 cells develop out of so-called naive T cells under the influence of a distinct cytokine combination (Figure 1). Increasing evidence suggests different T cell subpopulations differentiate to fulfil specialised tasks under specific pathogen-associated molecular patterns that create a distinct microenvironment. Such a scenario has recently been described by several groups for the homeostasis between Th17 and iTreg cells[ix,x]. A central role for regulating this homeostasis plays the commensal microflora of the gut that seems to enhance Th17 differentiation[xi,xii].

However, despite existence of distinct T cell subtypes, co-secretion of several lineage-indicating cytokines (so-called T cell plasticity) is a commonly observed phenomenon. T cells co-producing IFN-γ and IL-4 are called Th0, cells that co-produce IFN-γ and IL-17 are called Th1/IL-17 and Th2/IL-17 cells co-secrete IL-4 and IL-17.

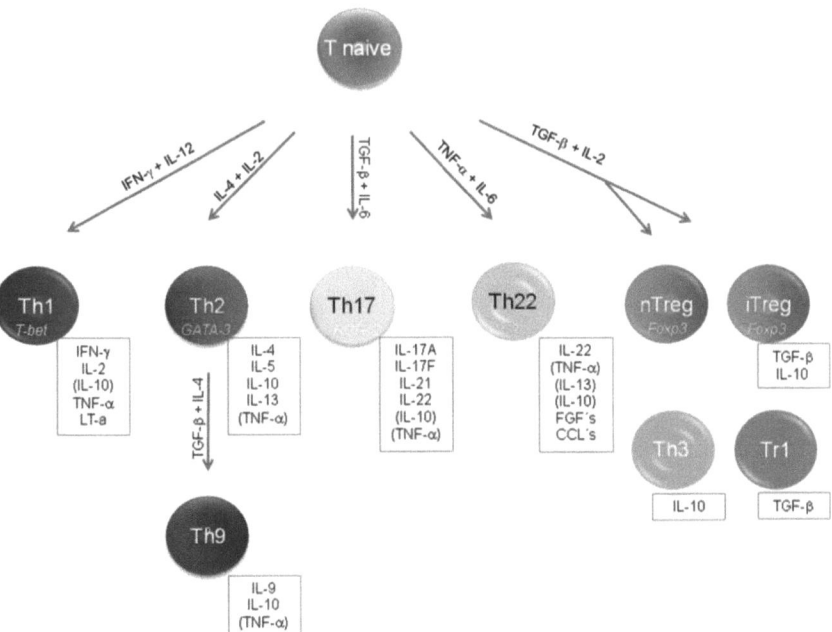

*Figure 1. Differentiation, key transcription factors (shown in italic font) and indicating effector cytokines of CD4+ T cell subsets identified so far.*


### 1.2 Non CD4+ T cell sources of IL-17 in the skin

Besides Th17, Th1/IL-17 and Th2/IL-17 cells, a broad variety of other leukocytes releases IL-17 upon adequate microenvironmental stimuli (Table 1).

All IL-17 producing leukocytes most likely share expression of the transcription factor RORc, the human analogue to mouse RORγt, shown to be essential for IL-17 production[xiii].

While human αβT cells (Th17; CD8+ IL-17 producing T cells) and NK cells (NKT) as sources of IL-17 have been extensively described in the last years, little is known about whether human γδT cells[xiv] and granulocytes produce this cytokine. In contrast, plenty of reports describe an essential role for IL-17 producing γδT cells in the initial phase of diverse infectious[xv,xvi,xvii] and immune-mediated[xviii,xix] disease models in the mouse system. Furthermore, indirect evidence exists that neutrophil granulocytes can produce IL-17 in mice, as SCID mice also develop neutrophilic responses associated with IL-17[xx].

However, given the quantitiy of CD8+, NKT and other non CD4+ T cells secreting IL-17 within the cellular infiltrate of inflamed skin, these cells contribute most likely marginally to the overall quantity of IL-17 in the skin. The main source of IL-17 in inflamed skin are CD4+ lymphocytes.

| Cell | Well characterised in human system | | | |
|---|---|---|---|---|
| | Other secreted factors | Evolution | Transcript. factor | Surface phenotype |
| Th17 | IL-21, IL-26, TNF-a, (IL-10), CCL20 | differentiation: naïve T cell +TGF-β/IL-1β/IL-6; IL-21; IL-23 | RORc | CD4+ CCR4+ CCR6+ CXCR3- CD161+ IL-23R+ |
| NKT | IFN-γ | | ROR | CD3+ CD56+ |
| LTi | TNF-α, Lymphotoxin | unknown (early NK cell?) | RORc | CD3- CD56- NKp44+ CD117+ CD127+ CD161+ |
| NK22 | TNF-α, Lymphotoxin, IL-26, leukaemia inhibitory factor | LTi cells (?) | RORc | CD3- CD56+ NKp44+ CD117+ CD127+ CD161+ |
| CD8+IL-17+ (human)/ Tnc17 | | Mouse: CD8+ T cell +TGF-β/IL-6 or +IL-1/IL-23 | Mouse: RORγt | CD3+ CD8+ CD45RO+ |
| Only single reports or described only in mice | | | | |
| γδT cell | | naïve T cell | | CD3+ CD4- CD8- CD27- CD25+ CD122- |
| T follicular helper cells | IL-21 | Naïve T cell +IL-21 +IL-6 +ICOSL | Unknown (BCL6?) | CD4+ ICOS+ CXCR5+ |
| Monocytes/ macrophages | | | RORγt | CD11b+ CD68+ |
| Neutrophil granulocyte | | | | |
| Paneth cells | TNF-a, GM-CSF, iNOS, Matrilysin | | | |

Table 1. Identified cellular sources of IL-17.

## 1.3 Th17 cells and known effects of IL-17 in the skin

Th17 cells have first been described in the year 2005 in the context of experimental autoimmune encephalitis[xxi]. Differentiation and expansion of Th17 cells are regulated stepwise by different cytokines (Figure 2): differentiation of Th17 cells out of naive T cells requires the cytokines TGF-β, IL-1β and IL-6[xxii,xxiii,xxiv]. A positive amplification loop of this process is created by ICOS-induced c-Maf via the production of IL-21[xxv]. In a third step, the cytokine IL-23 promotes a stable Th17 phenotype and expansion of Th17 cells[xxvi]. Discovery of IL-23 preceded the first description of Th17 cells[xxvii].

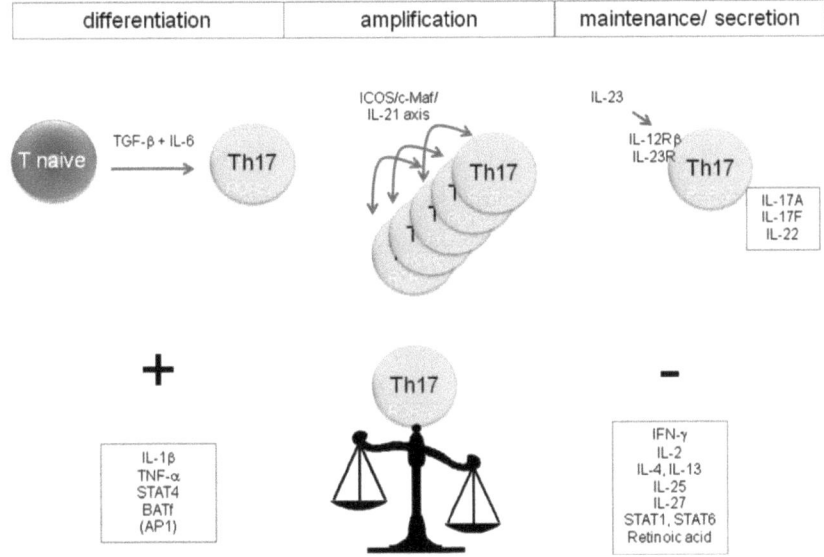

Figure 2. Regulation of T helper 17 cells.

Th17 cells are characterised by the production of IL-17A, IL-17F, IL-21, IL-22, IL-26 and the chemokine CCL20, which recruits CCR6+ cells[iv]. Th17 cells in turn express CCR6[xxviii]. A second recently described surface marker for Th17 cells is CD161, a molecule previously described to be expressed on Natural Killer cells[xxix,xxx].

Concerning effector functions of Th17 cells, increasing evidence suggests a strong pro-inflammatory role in several human diseases. Th17 cells are associated with autoimmune diseases like rheumatoid arthritis, multiple sclerosis and inflammatory bowel disease on the one and defence against several bacteria and fungi on the other hand[xxxi].

First evidence that IL-17 could be involved in host defence against *Candida* was given by Huang et al in 2004, showing that mice lacking IL-17 suffered from severed *Candida* infections[xxxii]. An association between *Candida* and Th17 cells was demonstrated both in the mouse and the human system in 2007[xxxiii,xxxiv]. Recently, IL-17 was identified as the main cytokine responsible for oral Candidiasis[xxxv].

Apart from *Candida albicans*, also other pathogens are related to a Th17 immune response. Among these are the bacteria *Propionibacterium acnes*, *Citrobacter rodentium*, *Klebsiella pneumoniae*, *Bacteroides* and *Borrelia* spp. and *Mycobacterium tuberculosis*xxxi.

A main pathway for antimicrobial effector functions of Th17 cells in the skin is through induction of innate immunity. IL-17 induces secretion of IL-8 in human keratinocytes, which represents a strong stimulus for migration of neutrophil granulocytes[xxxvi,xxxvii]. Furthermore, IL-17 and IL-22 induce secretion of antimicrobial peptides, the so called defensins, by human keratinocytes[xxxviii]. Defensins are critical for killing microorganisms[xxxix], and they induce migration of CCR6+ cells[xl], thus opening a pro-inflammatory circle by recruiting more Th17 cells into the skin.

## 1.4 The skin as a first-line defence organ of the organism

Epithelial cells build the interface between the human organism and its environment. Besides this mechanical protection that is warranted by continuous regeneration of the epithelial layer from the basal membrane, keratinocytes as main component of the human skin secrete an arsenal of immune-mediating cytokines and chemokines (Figure 3).

*Keratinocytes contribute to the inflammatory reaction*

To guarantee an adequate response, keratinocytes express a variety of sensing structures to detect microbial danger signals. Among these so-called "pattern recognition receptors", toll-like receptors (TLR) binding to bacterial, fungal or viral structures play a central role. Human keratinocytes express TLR 1-6, 9 and 10; however, only 3,4,5 and 9 seem to be functional[xli].

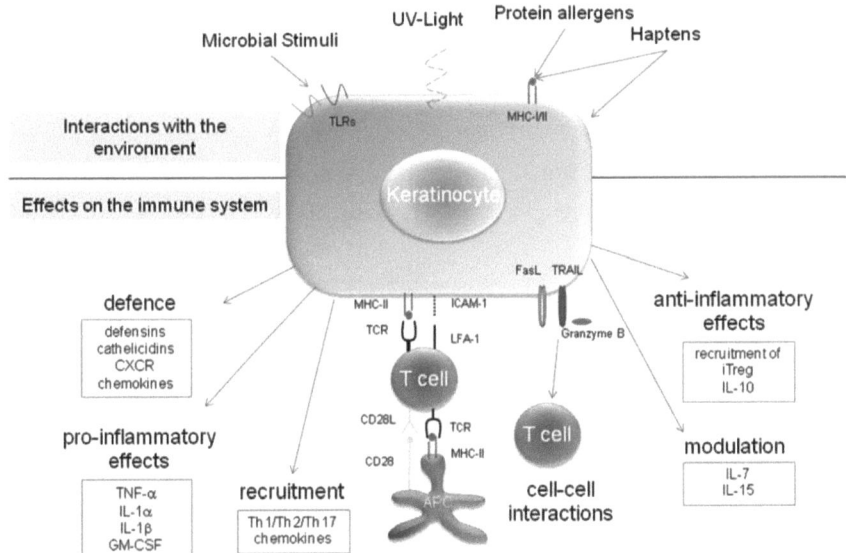

Figure 3. Human keratinocytes orchestrate innate and adaptive immunity in response to a wide range of external signals.

TLR-mediated activation of keratinocytes results in production of antimicrobial peptides, the so-called defensins and cathelicidins. Besides these direct antimicrobial effects that allow a control of skin colonization under normal conditions[xlii], keratinocytes recruit non-resident immune cells to sites of infection by secretion of a variety of chemokines[xli].

However, not only microbial stimuli activate keratinocytes. It has been shown that small molecules like haptens, that can elicit allergic reactions after binding to self-proteins, induce a pro-inflammatory response in keratinocytes that results in upregulation of ICAM-1, IL-1α, IL-1β, IL-1RA, TNF-α, CCL2 and CCL5[xliii].

As well as to external stimuli, keratinocytes respond to stimuli of the immune system. They constitutively express the receptor for IFN-γ. Binding of IFN-γ to keratinocytes induces expression of surface molecules (ICAM-1, HLA-ABC, HLA-DR, CD40), secretion of cytokines like IL-1, IL-18, IL-6, IL-15, GM-CSF, TNF-α, TGF-β and chemokines (CCL2, CCL3, CCL4, CCL5, CCL18, CCL22, CXCL8 und CX3CR ligands)[xliv,xlv]. Thus keratinocytes do not only contribute to a pro-inflammatory microenvironment, they also recruit additional immune cells.

Among recruited immune cells are neutrophil granulocytes via secretion of CXCL-8, CXCL-1, CCL-20 and IL-18[xlvi,xlvii], and various T cells. T cells expressing the skin homing molecule CCR10 are recruited via expression of CCL-27[xlviii], CXCR3+ Th1 cells via CXCL-9, CXCL-10 and CXCL-11, and CCR4+ Th2 cells via CCL-17 and CCL-22[xlix].

Interestingly, keratinocytes do not only recruit pro-inflammatory effector T cells, but also naturally occuring CD4$^+$CD25$^+$FoxP3$^+$ regulatory T cells or IL-10 producing Tr1 cells, especially via secretion ot CCL-1[l]. Thus keratinocytes do not only aggravate an inflammatory reaction, but also contribute to its limitation.

*Keratinocytes as target cells in inflammation*

Besides their role as active mediators of the immune reaction in the skin, keratinocytes are central target cells in the pathophysiology of an eczematous reaction. Upon stimulation with IFN-γ, keratoinocytes upregulate adhesion molecules like ICAM-1, HLA-ABC, HLA-DR and CD40 that allow a close morphological interaction with effector immune cells like T cells[li]. Such a close interaction leads to loss of epidermal integrity (cleavage of e-cadherin) and keratinocyte apoptosis, which results in edema and the clinical picture of eczema[lii,liii].

*Immune-modulatory capacity of keratinocytes*

Keratinocytes also express the T cell-modulating cytokines IL-12, IL-15 and IL-18. Secretion of IL-15 results in a extended life span especially of natural killer cells and some T cells in the skin and thus promotes a cytotoxic immune response[liv].

IL-12 on the other hand promotes the differentiation of type 1 T cells. Interestingly, among the two subunits of IL-12, the one shared with IL-23 (IL-12p35) is constitutively expressed in keratinocytes, while IL-12p40 is induced by e.g. contact allergens or haptens. This could explain type 1-dominated immune reactions during allergic contact dermatitis[lv]. IL-12 also influences the effects of IL-18; in presence of IL-12, IL-18 promotes a type I differentiation, while in absence of IL-12 a type 2 reaction is enhanced[lvi].

Taken together, keratinocytes are potent players in immunity against (extracellular) microorganisms by sensing external and internal danger signals and responding with an arsenal of cytokines, chemokines and antimicrobial peptides.

## 1.5 Chronic mucocutaneous candidiasis

*Candida albicans* is a ubiquitous, opportunistic yeast colonizing membranes of human skin and mucosal surfaces. The yeast causes infections (candidiasis) only, if the homeostasis between virulence of the microbe and resistance of the host immune system is disturbed. Chronic mucocutaneous Candidiasis (CMC) is a collective term for a complex group of disorders characterised by persistent or recurrent infections of the skin, nails and mucosal tissues. Patients with CMC rarely develop disseminated or systemic infections with *Candida*[lvii]. The first case of CMC was described by Thorpe and Handley in 1929[lviii], followed by other reports in the 1950s[lix,lx]. The term "chronic mucocutaneous candidiasis" was introduced in the late 1960s[lxi]. Today, CMC still is diagnosed clinically and by *in vitro* isolation and cultivation of *Candida* from smear tests. Additionally, diagnosis can be confirmed by mutational analysis in subgroups with known underlying genetical defects.

*Heterogeneity and prevalence of CMC*
The complex group of CMC syndromes can be subclassified according to distribution (local candidiasis versus generalized mucocutaneous candidiasis) and to underlying pathomechanism (primary versus secondary syndromes) (Table 2).
Notably, inherited CMC syndromes are often associated with autoimmune diseases of endocrine glands. This is the case in the autosomal-recessive "autoimmune polyendocrinopathy candidiasis ectodermal dystrophy syndrome" (APECED or APS-1)[lxii,lxiii], where monogenic defects in the autoimmune regulator gene (AIRE)lxiii,[lxiv,lxv] have been described, or in distinct syndromes of dominantly inherited CMC[lxvi] with endocrinopathies, where either the underlying genetic defect has been mapped on chromosome 2p[lxvii] or associations with a variant in the lymphoid protein tyrosine phosphatase have been reported[lxviii], respectively. For other primary forms of CMC the genetical basis is unknown. For all known mutations, however, the link between mutation and immune defect(s) remains unclear. In contrast, secondary CMC syndromes are usually the consequence of local or systemic immune-

suppression due to infections (especially AIDS, where candidiasis is of prognostic value[lxix]), reduced micro-perfusion in diabetes or immune-suppressive long-term medication. Another predisposing factor for secondary *Candida* infections is a disturbed microenvironment, e.g. after long-term antibiotic treatment or around dentures (Table 2).

| Name | Pathomechanism |
|---|---|
| Primary immunodeficiencies ||
| Autoimmune polyendocrinopathy candidiasis ectodermal dystrophy (APECED, also APS1) | mutation in AIRE gene; associated dysfunctions of endocrine glands |
| Autosomal-recessive CMC | mutation in PTPN22 gene; associated with autoimmune endocrinopathies and antibody deficiency |
| Autosomal-recessive CMC | unknown mutation(s) |
| Autosomal-dominant CMC | mutation mapped on chromosome 2p; associated with thyroid gland malfunction |
| Autosomal-dominant CMC | unknown mutation(s) |
| Autosomal-dominant hyper-IgE syndrome | mutation in STAT3 gene; associated with |
| Secondary CMC ||
| Chronic infection (HIV) | Immune-suppression |
| Metabolic disease (Diabetes, obesity) | |
| Long-term medication (corticosteroids, immunosuppressive drugs) | |
| Long-term antibiotic treatment | Alteration of local microenvironment |
| Denture | |

Table 2. Clinical syndromes underlying chronic mucocutaneous *Candidiasis*.

Concerning the prevalence of CMC syndromes, only data on APECED exist. APECED is most common in the small populations with high consanguinity of Iranian Jews (about 1:9.000)[lxx], Sardinians (1:14.400)[lxxi] and Finnish (1:25.000)[lxxii]. Both in the Jewish and the Finnish population old founder mutations responsible for almost all cases were detected[lxxiii]. Prevalence in Norway is estimated around 1:90.000[lxxiv]. In other parts of the world only sporadic cases of APECED have been reported. Similarly, no information is available on how frequent (or, rather orphan) non-APECED CMC syndromes are.

*Pathogenesis of CMC*

Defence against *Candida* requires an orchestrated immune response involving both innate and adaptive mechanisms. Though the pathogenesis of CMC is complex and may be heterogeneous, increasing evidence suggests that an altered T cell cytokine secretion is a central event.

In contrast, innate immunity generally seems functional in CMC patients[lxxv]. However, single reports exist demonstrating defects in innate immunity also. This is true for phagocytic cells such as neutrophil granulocytes, where a serum-dependent functional defect has been published[lxxvi]. However, recent studies indicate a normal candidicidal capacity and migratory behaviour of neutrophils in CMC patients[lxxvii,lxxviii]. A subtle impairment in activation and migration of other phagocytic cells such as macrophages or monocytes[lxxix] has also been reported in single CMC patients[lvii,lxxx], though these might be secondary effects due to an altered cytokine production. Furthermore, some studies suggest a defect in natural killer (NK) cells in CMC, either stating they were decreased[lxxxi] or functionally impaired[lxxxii].

There seems to be no general defect in humoral immunity also, as most CMC patients show normal serum concentrations of immunoglobulins and high titres of specific antibodies against *Candida* species[lvii,lxxxiii]. Again, within the heterogeneous group of CMC patients, a small subgroup seems to suffer from recurrent respiratory infections accompanied by deficiency of the IgG subclasses 2 and 4[lxxxiv].

However, protection against mucocutaneous *Candida* infections seems to rely mainly on cell-mediated immunity, in particular on T cells. Evidence for that hypothesis is given by the fact that patients lacking T cells due to a severe combined immunodeficiency or DiGeorge syndrome often suffer from oral candidiasis and *Candida* infections of skin and nail, but very rarely from systemic candidiasis[lxxxv]. The ability of T cells to proliferate to *Candida* antigen is discussed controversially: some studies describe a diminished proliferation both to *Candida* and to mitogens[lxxxvi], others state a specific defect in the proliferation to *Candida* or a normal T cell proliferation[lxxxvii]. Cytokine secretion of T cell subtypes rather than proliferation seems a more critical parameter in the pathogenesis of CMC. An impaired Th1 immune response leads to an increased susceptibility to severe *Candida* infections[lxxxvii] while reduction of IL-10 increases resistance against these infections[lxxxviii]. Furthermore, the T helper subset Th17 is essential in *Candida* resistance in mice and humans[lxxxix,xc,xci]. In fact, numerous studies show that CMC patients suffer from a deregulated T cell cytokine production, with a diminished production of type 1-cytokines[lxxvii,xcii,xciii,xciv] such as IFN-γ, IL-12 and IL-2 and an increased secretion of IL-10 or IL-4[xcv]. The observed effects, however, are not highly reproducible nor impressive. Whether deregulated T cell cytokine production is due to a direct T cell defect or a disturbed interaction with APC remains to be elucidated, as evidence exists that dendritic cells of CMC patients show an abnormal maturation[xcvi] while normal distribution of pattern recognition receptors[xcvii].

*Clinical course of CMC*

Impaired clearing of *Candida* is the basis for the main clinical symptoms of CMC, a chronic local inflammation, erosion/ulceration and hyperproliferation/ squamation of skin and mucosal epithelia that ranges from mild angular cheilitis to severely inflamed thick plaques and crusts (Figure 4). Predisposed areas are oral and oesophageal mucosa, trunk (especially axillary and vaginal region) and hands and nails (onychomycosis or candidal paronychia). Primary CMC syndromes usually show an early onset within the first years of life, while secondary CMC occurs in later life stages.

Clinically, CMC patients suffer from high psychological stress, dissatisfying aesthetical appearance and uncomfortable itch, burning sensations or pain. Furthermore, *Candida* plaques can cause severe clinical complications. Due to lesion expansion, local *Candida* plaques (*Candida granuloma*) can massively debilitate the use of hands. Another frequent and dangerous complication due to volume expansion and/or scarring after chronic inflammation is stricture of the oesophageus that has to be treated with balloon dilatation or stenting[xcviii]. A secondary consequence of chronic plaques in the gastrointestinal tract can be maldigestion or malabsorption with consecutive iron and vitamin deficiency or even excessive loss of weight and cachexia that requires intraveneous nutrition.

A third group of complications comprises metaplasia or neoplasia such as development of oral squamous cell carcinoma reported in several cases of severe

CMC[xcix,c,ci]. Potentially, neoplasia develops as a consequence of the chronic inflammation, as previously described for gastro-oesophageal reflux disease[cii] and cutaneous inflammation[ciii].

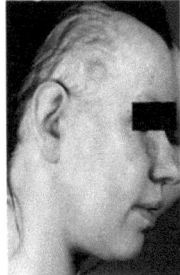 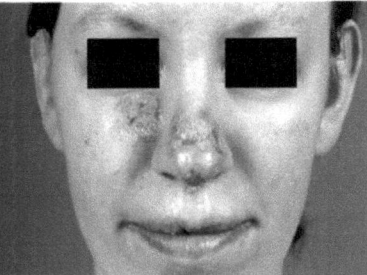 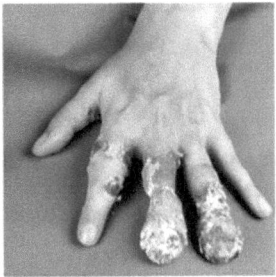

*Figure 4. Clinical manifestation of chronic mucocutaneous candidiasis at the skin.*

*Therapy of CMC*

Historically, CMC was treated with immune-stimulating or -restoring agents such as adoptive leukocyte transfer[civ] or thymus transplantation[cv]. After development of systemic anti-fungal drugs, however, long-term medication with azole antimycotics became the standard therapy of *Candida* infections[cvi] (Table 3). Azoles inhibit ergosterol synthesis, thereby acting static against *Candida*. Today fluconazole is recommended as first-line systemic drug in a dosage of 100-200mg/day. However, sensitivity against fluconazole often decreases over time[cvii]. Regular microbial sensitivity tests (antibiogram) of isolated *Candida* strains are therefore essential in the treatment of CMC. Itraconazole, voriconazole or posaconazole[cviii] are newer azole-antifungals that can substitute fluconazole.

Another class of systemic antifungal drugs applicable against *Candida* infections are the echinocandins[cix] caspofungin[cx], micafungin[cxi] and anidulafungin. They act against fungi by inhibition of glucan synthesis and therefore cell wall formation. The main disadvantage of echinocandins is lack of oral formulation. Echinocandins and azoles are comparably efficient against *Candida* infections. Though no long-term safety analyses are available, echinocandins seem relatively safe and show potential synergism with other antimycotics.

A third class of antifungal agents are polyenes that bind to ergosterol. The only polyene currently recommended for systemic anti-*Candida* treatment is amphotericin B; however, since it has to be administered intravenously and it shows severe side effects (in particular nephrotoxicity), amphotericin B has to be considered a third-line agent, although new lipid-associated formulations show lower toxic side effects[cxii]. Topical amphotericin B, however, is recommended as safe long-term treatment of local infections, as resistances are rarely observed.

| Class/ name | Recommended dosage | Additional information |
|---|---|---|
| Azoles (Triazoles) | | |
| fluconazole (first-line drug) | 100-200mg/day; systemic infections up to 800mg/day; pediatric 6-12mg/kg/day | Oral administration; Candida-static activity; sometimes resistances (esp. fluconazole); liver enzymes ↑, drug-drug-interactions |
| itraconazole | 200(-400)mg/day | |
| voriconazole | 400mg/day oral or 8mg/kg/day intravenous | |
| posaconazole | 600-800mg/day | |
| ravuconazole | No official recommendations yet (in clinical phase I and II studies) | |
| Echinocandins | | |
| caspofungin | 70mg/ first day, then 50mg/day (dose reduction in liver dysfunction) | Intravenous administration; Candidicidal activity; low side-effects (infusion reactions, liver enzymes ↑) |
| micafungin | 100-150mg/day; prophylaxis: 50mg/day | |
| anidulafungin | 200mg/first day, then 100mg/day | |
| Polyenes | | |
| local Amphotericin B | 2g/day | Local Candida infections (oral Candidiasis), safe and few resistances |
| liposomal amphotericin B | 3mg/kg/day | Intravenous administration; rarely infusion-related side effects and nephrotoxicity |

Table 3. Recommended anti-*Candida* drugs.

## 1.6 Atopy and atopic eczema

Atopic eczema (AE) is a chronic relapsing-remitting inflammatory skin disorder beginning mostly in early childhood. It is often associated with other atopic diseases such as allergic asthma and allergic rhinitis. The three atopic diseases can overlap or manifest at different life stages in the same individuum, which is called the atopic march[cxiii]. AE is highly pruritic and severely affects life quality of the single individual and it´s environment[cxiv]. The incidence of AE is continuously increasing[cxv,cxvi], which implies a high socioeconomic impact[cxvii].

The underlying pathogenesis of AE is a complex interaction of genetical predisposition and environmental factors (Figure 5). Defining hallmarks are the relapsing-remitting cutaneous inflammation, a disturbed epidermal barrier with a consecutive high transepidermal water-loss that results in dry skin, and a hyper-reactive immune system with IgE-mediated sensitisations against environmental allergens. Recently, a strong association with loss-of-function mutations in the gene filaggrin was reported[cxviii,cxix], which could be critically involved in the observed epidermal barrier dysfunction. Other known defects in building an accurate epidermal barrier in AE patients are mutations in the lipid metabolism that result in decreased ceramides and alterations in the SPINK5/LEKTI genes.

In between epidermal barrier dysfunction and immunological changes, psychosomatic aspects and physical factors determine the outcome of AE. Psychological pressure and stress worsen AE, and adjuvant mental relaxing techniques have been shown to improve skin inflammation and life quality of patients. As for physical factors, moderate doses of UV light improve cutaneous inflammation in AE, but extreme temperature and sweating have opponent effects. In general, AE patients take benefit from a rehabilitation sojourn in a low-allergen environment like the seaside or mountains, supporting a role both for physical and for allergic factors.

AE is often associated with type I (Th2-dominated) immune hyperreactivities mediated by allergen-specific IgE to common environmental or food allergenscxiv. The atopy patch test (APT) has been widely accepted as a model for allergen-specific induction of an acute atopic eczema by type I allergy inducing proteins such as pollen or house dust mite derived allergens[cxx]. AE and APT reactions share histological similarities with delayed type hypersensitivity responses, with the exception that in acute AE and APT lesions T helper 2 cytokines like IL-4, IL-5 and IL-13 are abundantly present[cxxi,cxxii].

Beyond deregulations within the adaptive branch of the immune system, innate immune responses are critical for the outcome of AE. Evidence exists that antimicrobial peptides, the so-called defensins, are reduced as compared to other immune mediated skin diseases like psoriasis, and this may be responsible for the high *Staph. aureus* skin colonisation[cxxiii].

*The role of skin-colonising microorganisms in atopic eczema*

More than 85% of AE patients are affected by skin colonisation with facultative pathogenic microbials like *Staph. aureus*[cxxiv]. Although *Staph. aureus* usually doesn't elicit imminent clinical signs of infection, its colonisation contributes to allergic sensitisation and inflammation. Infection of eczematous lesions with *Staph. aureus* is strongly associated with an increased disease severity[cxxv]. A suspected underlying mechanism is the frequent production of exotoxins by *Staph. aureus* species colonising AE skin[cxxv].

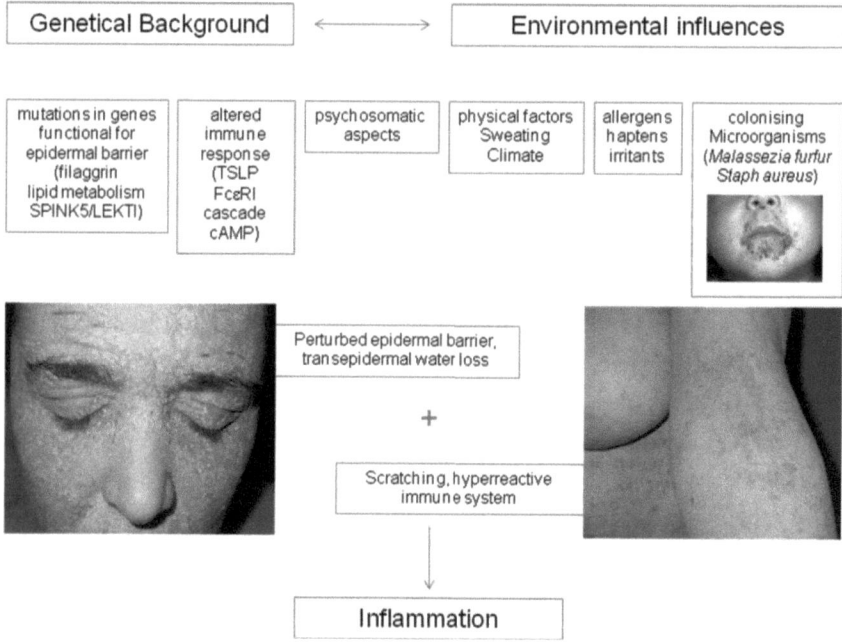

*Figure 5. The pathogenesis of atopic eczema is based upon complex interactions between genetical predispositions and environmental influences.*

These exotoxins stimulate T cells bearing particular T cell receptor Vβ chains regardless of their specificity and are therefore called superantigens[cxxvi]. Recently, the superantigen Staphylococcal enterotoxin B (SEB) was shown to enhance house dust mite-induced patch test reactions in AE patients, while only a minor proportion of AE patients developed an eczematous reaction to SEB alone. This study illustrates an enhancing role for bacterial-derived enterotoxins in the pathogenesis of AE[cxxvii].

## 2. Aim of the study

The aim of this study is to investigate the role of IL-17 in the first-line defence of the human organism against colonising and transient microorganisms. Since knock-out models are not available in the human system, two diseases are chosen that are frequently associated with an inability to clear skin infections – the orphan syndrome "chronic mucocutaneous candidiasis" and the common disease "atopic eczema".
The following questions will be addressed to gain insight in the role of IL-17:

1. Is the IL-17 pathway disturbed in patients with chronic mucocutaneous candidiasis?
   a) Do these patients have normal counts of IL-17 producing T cells in peripheral blood?
   b) Do T cells of CMC patients react with an adequate secretion of IL-17 in response to *Candida* antigen or to mitogen?
   c) Is there a defect in Th17 cell differentiation?
2. Why do patients with atopic eczema express only low amounts of antimicrobial peptides and consecutively suffer from chronic skin infections?
   a) Are IL-17+ T cells detectable in inflamed skin of AE patients and how is their pasticity?
   b) Can IL-17 secretion be efficiently triggered in T cells capable of IL-17 production?
   c) Is there an intrinsic defect in response to IL-17 in human keratinocytes?
   d) Does the Th2-dominated microenvironment of acute eczematous AE reactions inhibit IL-17 effects?

## 3. Materials and methods
### 3.1 Patients

For the characterisation of the T cell immune response of CMC patients, we included four patients with this orphan disease (Table 4).

| Initials | MG (I) | MF (I) | CB (I) | MS (III) |
|---|---|---|---|---|
| Age (years) | 27 | 37 | 48 | 8 |
| Sex | ♀ | ♀ | ♀ | ♂ |
| Clinical symptoms | Chronic oral, esophageal, vaginal and cutaneous candidiasis, paronychia | | | |
| Onset (at age) | Early (3) | Early (birth) | Early (birth) | Early (birth) |
| Endocrinology/ Immunology | Normal | Normal/ squamous cell carcinoma, ANA mildly positive | Normal | Morbus Addison, polyendocrinopathy syndrome/ normal |
| Laboratory markers | Iron deficiency anemia | CRP constantly elevated (3,5mg/dl) | Normal | Normal |
| Electrophoresis | Albumin 50,9%↓, γ-globulin 22,8%↑ | Albumin 56,9%↓, γ-globulin 22,0%↑ | Albumin 55,9%↓, γ-globulin 20,4%↑ | n.d. |
| Candida-Abs serum | IgG 258U/ml, IgM 1172U/ml | IgG <40U/ml, IgM <60U/ml | IgG 170U/ml, IgM <60U/ml | n.d. |
| Immunoglobulins serum | Normal, IgG4 0,20g/l↓ | Normal | IgG 1635mg/dl↑, IgA 940mg/dl↑ | n.d. |
| Phenotyping of T cells | Normal | Lymphopenia | Lymphopenia | n.d. |

Table 4. Clinical and laboratory characteristics of CMC patients included into the study.

Diagnosis was made clinically and confirmed by typical laboratory alterations. CMC patients were compared to four patients suffering from an (at the time of investigation) untreated *Candida* infection without any obvious immune suppression (Table 5) and to healthy volunteers (n=9).

| Initials | UD | WH | DU | LK |
|---|---|---|---|---|
| Age (years) | 47 | 65 | 39 | 51 |
| Sex | ♀ | ♂ | ♀ | ♀ |
| Clinical symptoms | Chronic paronychia and onychodystrophia | | | Vaginal Candidosis |
| Onset (at age) | Late (45) | Late (60) | Late (30) | Late (58) |
| Endocrinology/ Immunology | Normal | Normal | Normal | Diabetes mellitus/normal |
| Laboratory markers | Iron deficiency anemia | Normal | Normal | Normal |
| Electrophoresis | Albumin 63,2%→, γ-globulin 18,8%↑ | Albumin 60,0%→, γ-globulin 16,4%→ | n.d. | n.d. |
| Candida-Abs serum | IgG 52U/ml, IgM <60U/ml | IgG <40U/ml, IgM <60U/ml | n.d. | n.d. |
| Immunoglobulins serum | Normal | Normal | Normal | Normal |
| Phenotyping of T cells | Normal | Normal | Normal | Normal |

Table 5. *Clinical and laboratory characteristics of immune-competent patients with* chronic Candida *infection included into the study.*

Before blood was taken, each participant had given his informed consent. The study was approved by the ethical committee of the Technical University Munich, following the guidelines of the Helsinki declaration[cxxviii].

For the second model disease, three patients suffering from atopic eczema (AE) included into the study. Diagnosis was confirmed according to the criteria of Hanifin and Rajka[cxxix]. Furthermore, all patients suffered from a relevant allergy to house dust mite, as diagnosed with a positive prick test to *Dermatophagoides pteronyssinus* (Der p), RAST class ≥ 3 to Der p 1 and a positive Atopy Patch Test (APT) to Der p.

Before blood or skin samples were taken, each participant gave his informed consent. The study was approved by the ethical committee of the Istituto Dermopatico Dell'Immacolata.

## 3.2 Materials

*Biologic material*

| | |
|---|---|
| Albumin, bovine (BSA) | Sigma, Munich, A-8806 |
| *Candida albicans* | Sigma, Munich, IRMM354 |
| *Dermatophagoides pteronyssinus* | Indoor Biotechnology, UK |
|     Natural affinity purified | NA-DP1 |
|     Recombinant | RP-DP1 |
| Fetal bovine serum (FBS), | Perbio, Bonn |
| Human male AB Serum | Sigma, Munich, H-4522 |
| LPS | Sigma, Munich, L-4391 |
| Staphylococcal enterotoxin B | Sigma, Munich, S-4881 |

*Cell culture material*

| | |
|---|---|
| 96-well plates flat bottom sterile | Nunc, Roskilde, Denmark, 167008 |
| 96-well plates U-bottom sterile | Nunc, Roskilde, Denmark, 163320 |
| 96-well maxisorp plates flat bottom | Nunc, Roskilde, Denmark, 449824 |
| Clustertubes 1,2ml | Abgene, Surrey, UK, AB-0672 |
| Cryo tubes 1,8ml | Nunc, Roskilde, Denmark, 375418 |
| Eppendorf tubes | Eppendorf, Hamburg, 0030 015.002 |
| Falcon Polypropylen tubes | Becton Dickinson, NJ, USA |
|     15 ml/50 ml | 352070 / 2096 |
| Heat sealing paper ($\beta$-Counter) | Perkin Elmer, Rodgau-Jügesheim, 1450-467 |
| LS columns (MACS) | Miltenyi, Bergisch-Gladbach, 130-041-306 |
| Melti Lex TMA ($\beta$-Counter) | Perkin Elmer, Rodgau-Jügesheim, 1450-441 |

| | |
|---|---|
| Printed Filtermat A (β-Counter) | Perkin Elmer, Rodgau-Jügesheim, 1450-421 |
| Sterile filter units 500ml | Millipore, FCGVUO5RE |
| Surgical scissor Aesculap | Braun, Melsungen, BC107R |

*Chemicals*

| | |
|---|---|
| 2-Mercapto-Ethanol | Sigma, Munich, M-7522 |
| Adenine | Sigma, Munich, A-9795 |
| Antibiotic-Antimycotic Solution | PAA, Linz, Austria, P11-002 |
| Aqua ad injectabilia | Delta-Select, Pfullingen |
| CFSE | Molecular Probes, Leiden, Netherlands, C-1157 |
| Cholera toxin | Sigma, Munich, C-3012 |
| DMSO | Baker, Griesheim, 7157 |
| DMEM | Invitrogen, Paisley, UK, 41966-029 |
| DPBS Ca/Mg | Invitrogen, Paisley, UK, 14040174 |
| DPBS w/o Ca/Mg | Invitrogen, Paisley, UK, 14190094 |
| EDTA | Sigma, Munich, ED4SS |
| EDTA 0,5M | Invitrogen, Paisley, UK, 15575-020 |
| Epidermal growth factor (EGF) | Sigma, Munich, E-4127 |
| Gentamycin | Invitrogen, Paisley, UK, 15710049 |
| Glucose | Sigma, Munich, G-7528 |
| HAM's F12 | Sigma, Munich, N-6760 |
| HBSS w/o Ca/Mg | Invitrogen, Paisley, UK, 24020091 |
| Heparin 250.000U | Ratiopharm, Ulm, PZN-7833909 |
| Hydrocortisone | Sigma, Munich, H-0135 |
| Insulin | Sigma, Munich, I-1882 |
| Keratinocyte medium | Promocell, Wien, Austria, C-20211 |
| L-Glutamine | Invitrogen, Paisley, UK, 25030024 |
| Lymphoprep | Progen Biotechnik, Heidelberg, 111-4545 |
| Mitomycin C | Sigma, Munich, M-4287 |
| Nickel sulphate | Sigma, Munich, N-4882 |

| | |
|---|---|
| Non-essential amino acids | Invitrogen, Paisley, UK, 11140-35 |
| Penicillin-Streptomycin | Invitrogen, Paisley, UK, 15140130 |
| PHA (Lectin) | Sigma, Munich, L-9132 |
| Reverse transcriptase | Roche, Mannheim |
| RNA extraction buffer (PeqGold) | Peqlab, Erlangen |
| RPMI 1640 + L-Glutamine | Invitrogen, Paisley, UK, 31870-025 |
| Sodium pyruvate | Invitrogen, Paisley, UK, 11360-039 |
| SYBR green master mix | Bio-Rad, Munich, Germany |
| Transferrin | Sigma, Munich, T-5391 |
| Trypan blue 0,4% solution | Sigma, Munich, T-8154 |
| Trypsin 0,05% EDTA | Invitrogen, Paisley, UK, 2530054 |

*Cytokines and antibodies*

| | |
|---|---|
| anti-CCR4 PE | R&D systems, clone 205410 |
| anti-CCR6 PE | BD pharmigen, clone 11A9 |
| anti-CD14 FITC | BD bioscience, clone MφP9 |
| anti-CD1a FITC | BD pharmigen, clone HI149 |
| anti-CD28 | BD bioscience, clone 37.51 |
| anti-CD3 | BD bioscience, clone 145-2C11 |
| anti-CD4 PE | BD bioscience, clone SK3 |
| anti-CD4 FITC | BD bioscience, clone SK3 |
| anti-CD56 FITC | BD bioscience, clone NCAM16.2 |
| anti-CD8 PE | BD bioscience, clone SK1 |
| anti-CD8 FITC | BD pharmigen, clone RPA-T8 |
| anti-CD83 FITC | BD pharmigen, clone HB15e |
| anti-CD86 FITC | BD pharmigen, clone 2331FUN1 |
| anti-CXCR3 | R&D systems, clone 49801.111 |
| anti-HLA-DP | R&D systems, 347730 |
| anti-HLA-DQ | R&D systems, 347450 |
| anti-HLA-DR | R&D systems, 347360 |
| anti-IL10 PE | BD pharmigen, clone JES3-19F1 |
| anti-IL4 FITC | BD pharmigen, clone MP4-25D2 |
| anti-IFN-γ FITC | BD pharmigen, clone B27 |
| anti-IFN-γ APC | BD pharmigen, clone B27 |

| | |
|---|---|
| anti-TNF-α FITC | BD pharmigen, clone Mab11 |
| anti-IL22 PE | R&D systems, clone 142928 |
| anti-IL4 PE | R&D systems, clone 3007.11 |
| anti-IL-17 | R&D systems, clone AF-317 |
| anti-IL17A PE | eBioscience, clone SK3 |
| GM-CSF | Schering Plough |
| IFN-γ | BD bioscience, 554617 |
| IL-13 | R&D Systems, 213-IL-005 |
| IL-17 | R&D Systems, 317-ILB-050 |
| IL-1β | R&D systems, 201-LB-005 |
| IL-2 | Novartis, Munich |
| IL-23 | R&D Systems, 1290-IL-010 |
| IL-4 | R&D Systems, 204-IL-010 |
| IL-6 | R&D Systems, 206-IL-010 |

*ELISA systems and kits*

| | |
|---|---|
| HBD-2 | Phoenix pharmaceuticals |
| Iotest Beta Mark Repertoire Kit | Beckman Coulter |
| IFN-γ duoset | R&D systems, DY285 |
| IL-4 duoset | R&D systems, DY204 |
| IL-10 duoset | R&D systems, DY217B |
| IL-13 duoset | R&D systems, DY213 |
| IL-17 duoset | R&D systems, DY317 |
| IL-22 duoset | R&D systems, DY782 |
| TNF-α duoset | R&D systems, DY210 |

*Machines*

| | |
|---|---|
| Camera | WILD MPS 52, Leitz-Leica, Wetzlar |
| Centrifuge "Biofuge 13" | Heraeus, Hanau |
| Centrifuge "Megafuge 1.0R" | Heraeus, Hanau |
| FACS"Calibur" | Becton Dickinson, Heidelberg |
| FACS"Aria" | Becton Dickinson, Heidelberg |
| Homogeniser | Ultra Turrax T 25 basic, IKA Werke, Staufen |

| | |
|---|---|
| Light microscope | Aristoplan, Leitz-Leica, Wetzlar |
| Light microscope | Axiovert 25, Zeiss, Jena |
| Multi-channel pipette | Eppendorf, Hamburg |
| Pipettes „reference" | Eppendorf, Hamburg |
| Precise weighing machince | MC1 Research, Sartorius, Göttingen |
| Real-time PCR "ABI Prism 7000" | Applied biosystems, Foster City, CA |
| Shaker | Titramax 100, Heidolph, Schwabach |
| Weighing machine | MC1Labor, Sartorius, Göttingen |
| Water bath „type 1003" | GFL, Burgwedel |

*Used media*

3T3-medium

    DMEM, 10% FCS (30min at 56° C de-activated), 5ml Pen/Strept.

    Stored at 4-8°C, used within 10 days

Antibiotic-antimycotic solution for keratinocyte isolation

    solution I: 500ml DMEM, 15ml gentamycin, 20ml *Antibiotic-Antimycotic solution*

        solution II: 250ml Lösung I + 250ml DMEM

        solution III: 250ml MEM + 2,5ml *Antibiotic-Antimycoticsolution*

    Sterile filtered, stored at -20°C

Feeder-/ keratinocyte medium

    300ml DMEM, 150ml HAM´s F12, 10ml glutamin, 50ml Hyclone II FCS, 5ml senicillin/streptomycin, 1ml adenin (= 1g), 1ml hydrocortisone (= 1g), 0,5ml Trijodthyronine (= 1mg), 0,5ml Cholera toxin (= 1mg), 0,5ml EGF (Epidermal Growth Factor; = 0,1mg), 0,5ml insulin (= 100mg), 0,5ml transferrin (= 10mg)

    Sterile filtered, stored at 4°C, used within 14 days

Mitomycin solution

    Mitomycin C 2mg

    Stock solution (500µg/ml): dissolved in 4ml DPBS ($+Ca^{2+}/Mg^{2+}$).

    Stored at 4°C in the dark

    Ready-to-use solution: 2% (diluted in RPMI 1640) Medium sterile filtered

MACS buffer
> 500ml DPBS Dulbecco´s w/o Ca/Mg, w/o Sodium bicarbonate, 2ml EDTA (2mM, diluted from Invitrogen 0,5M EDTA, pH 8,0), 2,5g bovine serum albumin (0,5%)
> Sterile filtered, oscillated in ultrasound-bath before usage for 15min


Proliferation medium (RPMI complete 5% human serum)
> 450ml RPMI 1640 Medium with L-Glutamin (Gibco™, Lot No. 3063498), 28ml human serum, 5ml L-glutamin, 5,6ml non-essential amino acids, 5,6ml sodium pyruvate, 500µl 50mM 2-Mercapto-ethanol
> Sterile filtered, stored at 4°C, used within 7 days

EBV-Medium
> RPMI complete with 50ml FCS (=10%), no human serum

cloning medium
> RPMI complete with 25ml human serum (= 5%), 50ml FCS (30min at 56°C heat inactivated) (= 10%), 5ml *antibiotic-antimycotic solution*
> Sterile filtered, stored at 4°C, used within 7 days


## 3.3 Methods

**Methods for part A (Th17 deficiency in CMC patients)**

*Isolation of peripheral blood mononuclear cells (PBMC)*

For isolation of PBMC, venous blood was taken from the forearm of patients and healthy volunteers in a syringe containing heparin. Blood was diluted 1:2 in DPBS and then transferred to a density gradient (15ml Lymphoprep medium in a 50ml tube) and centrifuged at 470xg for 20 minutes without brake. After centrifugation, the separated band of PBMC was recovered with a 5ml pipette and washed three times in DPBS (409xg for 15 minutes, then two times 301xg for 10 minutes). An aliquot of PBMC was counted in a 0,5% Trypan blue solution, then the rest of the PBMC was resuspended in proliferation medium in a defined concentration prior the experiments.

*Separation of CD4+ and CD8+ T cells*

For some experiments, CD4+ and CD8+ T cells were purified from isolated PBMC using magnetic bead labeling. 20µl anti-CD4 or anti-CD8 microbeads and 80µl MACS buffer per $10^7$ PBMC were incubated for 15 minutes at 4° C and separated by positive selection through a magnetic column. Cells were then washed, counted and resuspended in proliferation medium.

*Stimulation and co-culture experiments*

PBMC were cultured in flat-bottom 96well plates ($3,5*10^5$/well) and stimulated with either *Candida* antigen (100µg/ml), Phytohemagglutinin (PHA) (10µg/ml) or coated antiCD3/antiCD28 antibodies. For isolation of total RNA PBMC were stimulated for 6 hours, for quantification of secreted cytokines into supernatant by ELISA PBMC were stimulated for 60 hours.

*Flow cytometry analysis*

PBMC were stimulated with PMA (20 ng/ml) and ionomycin (1ng/ml) for 6 hours and examined for intracellular cytokine accumulation.

To prevent cytokine secretion, the stimulation was performed in the presence of Monensin (from the beginning) and Brefeldin A (10 g/ml) was added for the final 4 hours. T cells were fixed (2% paraformaldehyde), permeabilized (0,5% saponin), and stained with PE-conjugated anti human IL-17 antibody or isotype-matched control antibody. Acquisition and analysis was done using a FACS Calibur.

*Enzyme-linked immunosorbent assay (ELISA)*

Concentrations of IFN-$\gamma$, IL-4, IL-10, IL-17, IL-22, IL-1$\beta$, and IL-6 in cell-free culture supernatant were quantified using commercially available sandwich ELISA kits.

*RNA isolation and Real time PCR*

Total mRNA from stimulated PBMC was extracted using PeqGold RNA extraction buffer. RNA was reverse transcribed using oligo(dT) primers and AMV reverse transcriptase. PCR reactions were performed with synthetic oligonucleotides reacting specifically against IL-1β, IL-6, IL-17A, IL-17F, IL-22, and IL-23A (sequences see Table 6). SYBR green mastermix was added.

| Name of gene | Sequence |
| --- | --- |
| IL-1β | forward 5'-TTC GAC ACA TGG GAT AAC GA-3' |
| | reverse 5'-TCT TTC AAC ACG CAG GAC AG-3' |
| IL-6 | forward 5'-ATG CAA TAA CCA CCC CTG AC-3' |
| | reverse 5'-GAG GTG CCC ATG CTA CAT TT-3' |
| IL-17A | forward: 5'-CTC GAT TTC ACA TGC CTT CA-3' |
| | reverse 5'-GAG GGG CCT TAA TCT CCA AA-3' |
| IL-17F | forward 5'-AGT TGG AGA AGG TGC TGG TG-3' |
| | reverse 5'-CCA TCC GTG CAG GTC TTA TT-3' |
| IL-22 | forward 5'-GAG GAA TGT GCA AAA GCT GA-3' |
| | reverse 5'-GCT TTG GGG CAT CTA ATT GT-3' |
| IL-23A | forward 5'-CAG TTC TGC TTG CAA AGG AT-3' |
| | reverse 5'-ATC TGC TGA GTC TCC CAG TG-3' |

*Table 6. Real-time PCR primers used in the study. Primer sequences were obtained from www.realtimeprimers.com*

PCR reactions were run on an ABI Prism 7000 Sequence Detection System using the following program: 10 min at 94°C followed by 45 cycles of 15 s at 95°C, and 60 s at 58°C. 18 s RNA served as housekeeping gene.

*Statistical analysis*
Statistical analysis was performed by the software programme SPSS 14.0. Differences between the CMC group and healthy controls or immune competent *Candida*-infected patients were analysed using Mann-Whitney-U test. Statistically significant differences between CMC patients and controls were defined as p<0,05.

## Methods for part B (IL-17 in AE patients)
*Isolation and characterisation of skin-derived T cells*
To analyse T cells at clonal level, T cells derived from positive Atopy Patch Tests were cloned by limiting dilution.
Atopy Patch Tests containing house dust mite (*Dermatophagoides pteronyssinus*, Der p) were applied in large Finn chambers (11 mm in diameter) on the back of the

patients using petrolatum as carrier. Petrolatum alone served as negative control. After 48 hours the Finn chambers were removed and tested areas were marked. The test was evaluated after 48 and 72 hours. Positive reactions were classified according to the European Task Force on Atopic Dermatitis (ETFAD) 2000 reading key[cxxx].

T cells were then isolated from positive patch test lesions (Figure 6). For that purpose, punch biopsy specimens (4mm in diameter) were taken from positive APT reactions from the centre of the patch test areas after local anaesthesia had been administered (1% lidocaine). Biopsies were immediately cultured in proliferation medium containing 60 IU/ml recombinant IL-2).

After three days, half the medium was replaced by fresh medium containing IL-2. After seven days, migrated cells were collected and cloned by limiting dilution. T cells were counted and diluted to a concentration of 0,6 cells/well in 96-well U-bottom microplates in cloning medium on a feeder layer (450.000/well) of irradiated PBMC, 30U/ml IL-2 and 1% PHA. Fresh medium containing IL-2 was added three times a week and clones were restimulated using irradiated feeder PBMC every three to four weeks.

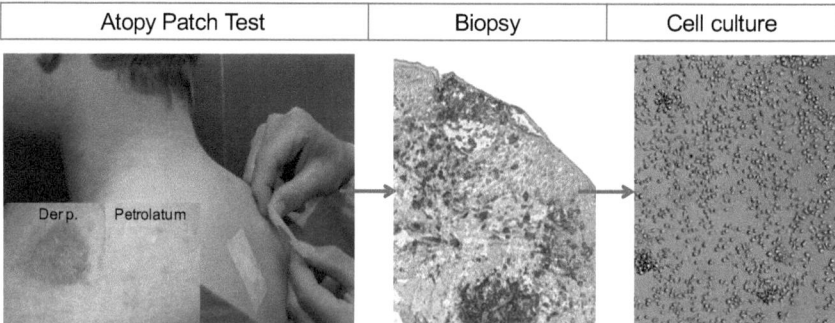

*Figure 6. Isolation of T cells from inflammatory skin reactions. Acute eczematous reactions were induced in sensitized patients (APT), biopsied and migrated cells were cultured in T cell medium.*

Growing T cell clones were expanded and characterised regarding cytokine secretion profile and Der p 1 reactivity. Clones were stimulated with either coated anti-CD3/anti-CD28 or autologous dendritic cells and Der p 1, respectively. After 48 hours, cell-free supernatant was obtained and the content of TNF-$\alpha$, IFN-$\gamma$, IL-4, IL-10, IL-13, IL-17 and IL-22 was determined by ELISA. Proliferation was investigated using the $^3$H-Thymidine assay. After 48 hour stimulation, 2µCi/ml $^3$H-thymidine was added to the cultures for additional 12 hours. Cells were then harvested on a filter, dried and afterwards reactivity was measured in a $\beta$-counter. In this setting, the amount of incorporated thymidine directly correlates with the proliferation of the T cells.

*Definition of T cell subtype*

T cell clones were classified according to their relative cytokine secretion into supernatant of the lead cytokines IFN-$\gamma$ (Th1), IL-4 (Th2), IL-10 (Th3), IL-17 (Th17), and IL-22 (Th22) after 48 hour stimulation with anti-CD3/anti-CD28. Table 6 illustrates the relative cytokine profile of each T cell population.

|  | IFN-$\gamma$ | IL-4 | IL-10 | IL-17 | IL-22 |
|---|---|---|---|---|---|
| Th1 | >80% | <5% | <20% | <5% | <20% |
| Th2 | <20% | >50% | <50% | <5% | <20% |
| Th3 | <20% | <5% | >80% | <5% | <20% |
| Th17 | <20% | <5% | <20% | >50% | <50% |
| Th22 | <20% | <5% | <20% | <5% | >80% |

*Table 7. Definition of T cell subpopulations according to their relative cytokine secretion of lineage-indicating cytokines.*

*Isolation and generation of antigen-presenting cells (APC)*

Dendritic cells were generated from CD14+ monocytes[25]. CD14+ monocytes isolated by magnetic labelling and positive selection out of PBMC were cultured in RPMI 1640 supplemented with 2 mM L-glutamine, 0.5 mM 2-Mercaptoethanol, 20 µg/ml gentamycin 10% FBS, 50 U/ml human rGM-CSF and 200 U/ml human rIL-4 (complete DC medium) with a complete change of medium after 3 days. At day 5, a part of the cells was stimulated with 50µg/ml LPS for 24 hours. Immediately before coculture experiments, cells were harvested and characterized for maturation markers (CD83, CD86, HLA-DR) and CD1a using flow cytometry.

*Suspension and culture of primary human keratinocytes*
To establish an autologous model of eczema, after isolating T cell clones keratinocytes were isolated from the same individuals using the method of suction blister[26]. Blisters were induced by generating a vacuum on normal skin of the forearms. Epidermal sheets were obtained from blister roofs, treated with 0.05% trypsin (Invitrogen) to obtain single-cell suspension and seeded on a feeder layer of irradiated 3T3/J2 fibroblasts in modified Green's medium. At 70–80% confluence, keratinocytes were detached with 0.05% trypsin, aliquoted, and cryopreserved in liquid nitrogen. Keratinocytes of second and third passage were used in experiments.

*Stimulation and co-culture experiments*
$10^5$ T cells and between 100 and 10000 immature or mature DC were co-cultured in flat-bottom 96well plates in RPMI complete 5% human serum for 36 hours with 5μg/ml Der p 1, 10μg/ml PMA/ 1μg/ml ionomycine, 5μg/ml SEB or full medium as negative control, respectively. Cell-free supernatant was obtained and T cell proliferation was analysed by $^3$H thymidine incorporation as described above.

*Patch testing of house dust mite and SEB* in vivo
To investigate the SEB/IL-17/HBD-2 axis *in vivo*, commercially available Der p was applied at the two forearms of an AE patient. 36 hours after allergen application, 50μg/cm² SEB was added on one forearm. Sixty hours after allergen application, epidermal sheets and blister fluid of induced eczematous reactions were obtained by the method of suction blister. RNA was prepared from epidermal roofs as described above, suction blister fluid was analysed using the Luminex method and by HBD-2 ELISA as described above (Figure 7).

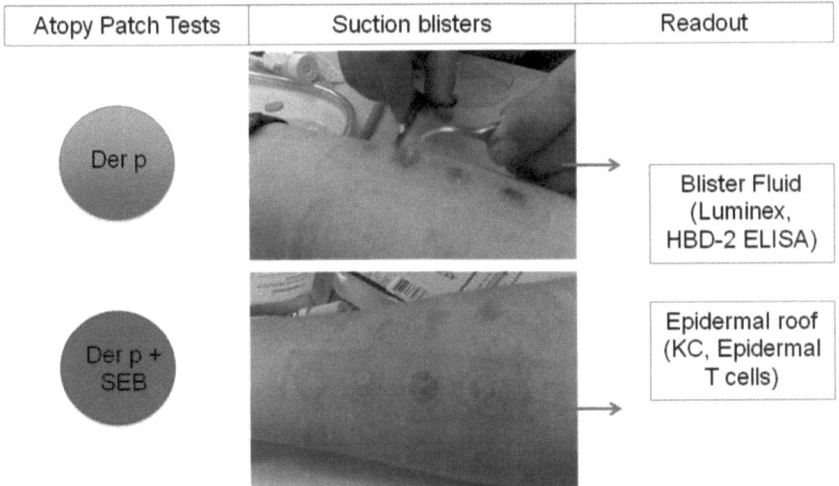

*Figure 7. Application of house dust mite and SEB in vivo.*


*Flow cytometry analysis*

T cell receptor Vβ repertoire of selected T cell clones was analysed using the "Iotest Beta Mark Repertoire Kit" following the instructions of the manufacturer.

Surface marker staining of skin-derived T cell lines or resting T cell clones was performed with 105 T cells for 15 mintes on ice and in the dark. After the incubation period, cells were washed in FACS buffer and acquisition was performed using a FACS calibur.

For intracellular cytokine analyses, skin-derived T cell lines or resting T cell clones were stimulated with PMA (20 ng/ml) and ionomycin (1ng/ml) for 6 hours. To prevent cytokine secretion, Monensin was added in the beginning and Brefeldin A (10 g/ml) was added for the final 4 hours of stimulation. T cells were then fixed (2% paraformaldehyde), permeabilized (0,5% saponin), and stained with conjugated antibodies (IFN-γ, IL-4, IL-17, IL-22, TNF-α) or isotype-matched control antibodies. Acquisition and analysis was done using a FACS Calibur.

*Enzyme-linked immunosorbent assay (ELISA)*

Concentrations of IFN-γ, IL-4, IL-10, IL-13, IL-17, IL-22, TNF-α and human β-defensin2 in cell-free culture supernatant were quantified using commercially available sandwich ELISA kits of indicated companies.

*RNA isolation and Real time PCR*

Total cellular mRNA was extracted from stimulated keratinocytes employing the phenol/chloroform method. RNA was then reverse transcribed using oligo(dT) primers and AMV reverse transcriptase. PCR reactions were performed with synthetic oligonucleotides reacting specifically against HBD-2 (sequences see Table 8). SYBR green mastermix was added.

| Name of gene | Sequence |
| --- | --- |
| HBD-2 | forward: 5'-TCCTCTCGTTCCTCTTCATATT-3' |
|  | reverse: 5'-TTAAGGCAGGTAACAGGATCGC-3' |

Table 8. *Real-time PCR primers used in the study. Primer sequences were obtained from www.realtimeprimers.com*

PCR reactions were run on an ABI Prism 7000 Sequence Detection System using the following program: 10 min at 94°C followed by 45 cycles of 15 s at 95°C, and 60 s at 58°C. GAPDH was housekeeping gene.

*Statistical analysis*

Differences in cytokine production and secretion in T cell clones and keratinocytes were analysed using a two-tailed Student's t-test. Statistically significant differences were defined as $p<0,05$.

## 4. Results
### 4.1 CMC patients suffer from an impaired secretion of IL-17 and IL-22

*PBMC of CMC patients show a strong decrease in IL-17 and IL-22 secretion upon stimulation*

Since a T cellular immune defect was hypothesised by us and others in patients with CMC, we stimulated PBMC of four CMC patients with *Candida albicans* as well as with mitogen (Phythemagglutinin). Immune competent healthy volunteers (n=9) and immune competent patients with an acute *Candida*-infection (n=4) served as controls. As a first step, we investigated the cytokine induction in PBMC at genetic level. For that purpose, we stimulated PBMC for 12 hours and then isolated total mRNA, reverse transcribed and amplified it in real time PCR and compared the cytokine mRNA level with that of un-stimulated PBMC (Figure 8).

Indeed we observed that IL-17F and IL-22 were significantly induced in PBMC of healthy (non-*Candida* infected) controls and immune competent Candidiasis patients, whereas CMC patients failed to upregulate the expression of these cytokines on mRNA level (Figure 8). Differences in upregulation of IL-17 and IL-22 mRNA in response to both *Candida albicans* and to PHA were significant ($p > 0,05$) between CMC patients and both immune competent control groups, while no significant differences were observed between healthy volunteers and Candidiasis patients.

The impaired upregulation of IL-17 and IL-22 mRNA was irrespective of the stimulus, as both specific stimulation with *Candida albicans* and mitogenic stimulation with PHA did neither induce IL-17 nor IL-22 (Figure 8). IL-17A was not upregulated in CMC patients and healthy controls in the monitored time course (data not shown).

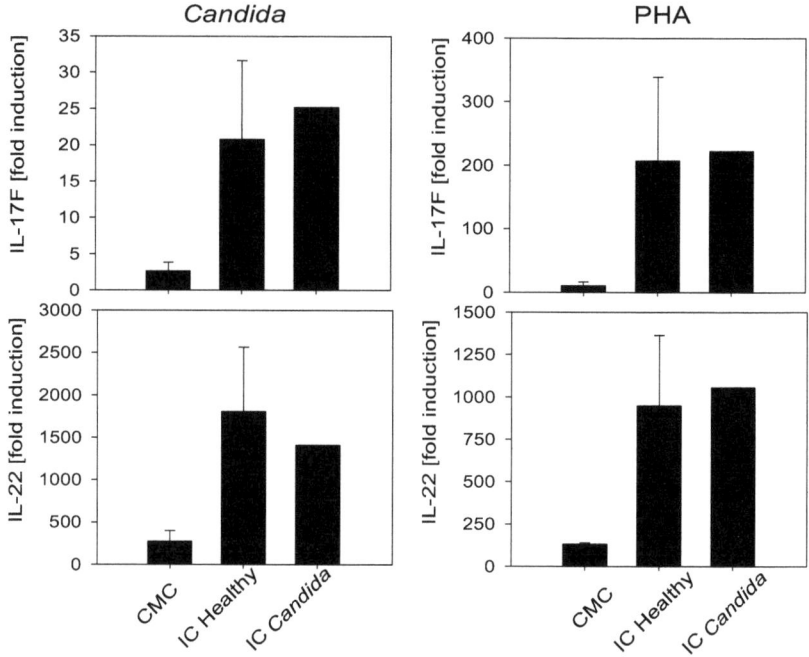

*Figure 8. CMC patients fail to upregulate IL-17 and IL-22 mRNA. Upregulation of IL-17 (upper panel) and IL-22 (lower panel) is given at the y-axis. Shown is the mean of three independent experiments (3 CMC patients, 4 healthy controls, 1 Candidiasis patient in total). Error bars indicate mean +/- SEM. (CMC: chronic mucocutaneous candidasis; IC healthy: immune competent volunteers; IC Candida: immune competent Candidiasis patients)*

An impaired IL-17 and IL-22 immune response in CMC patients as observed on transcriptional level was confirmed at secretion level of proteins. PBMC of CMC patients released very low amounts of IL-17A/F and IL-22 into culture supernatant after stimulation with either *Candida albicans* or PHA as measured by ELISA after 72 hours stimulation (Figure 9). In contrast, healthy volunteers secreted significantly higher amounts of Il-17A/F and IL-22. Even more impressive was the production of IL-17 and IL-22 in immune competent patients with current *Candida* infection that was significantly higher than that of CMC patients and of healthy volunteers (Figure 9).

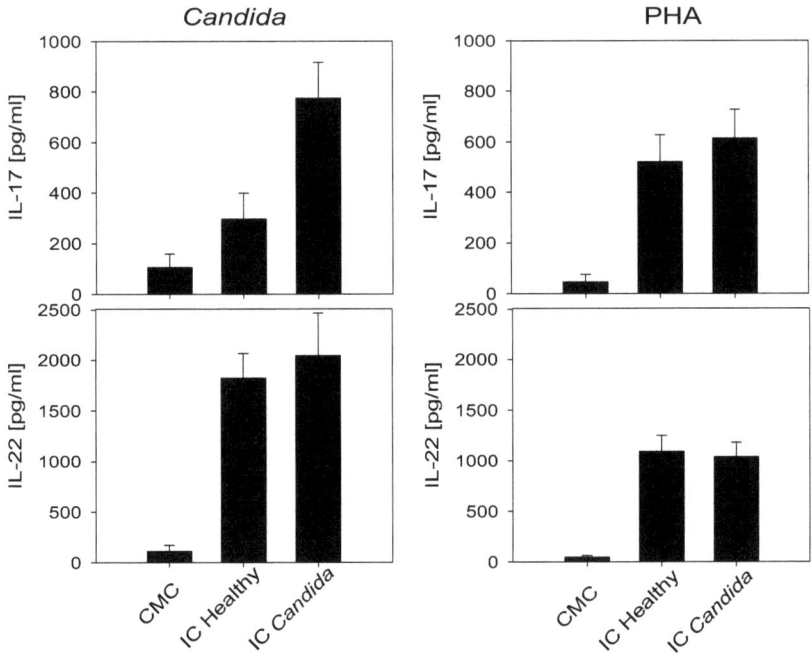

*Figure 9. Impaired IL-17 and IL-22 secretion in PBMC of CMC patients. Secretion of IL-17 (upper panel) and IL-22 (lower panel) is given at the y-axis. Shown is the mean of five independent experiments (4 CMC patients, 9 healthy controls, 4 Candidiasis patients in total). Error bars indicate mean +/- SEM. (CMC: chronic mucocutaneous candidasis; IC healthy: immune competent volunteers; IC Candida: immune competent Candidiasis patients)*

In the next step, we wanted to analyse whether the observed diminished secretion of IL-17 and IL-22 in PBMC was the consequence of a direct T cell defect or of an impaired antigen presentation by dendritic cells (DC). We therefore stimulated PBMC from CMC patients and immune competent controls with anti-CD3/anti-CD28, thus directly stimulating the T cells. Again, we observed a clearly diminished induction at mRNA level and secretion at protein level in CMC patients (Figure 10). This finding points to a defect in the T cell compartment rather than in antigen-presentation or absent APC-derived signals.

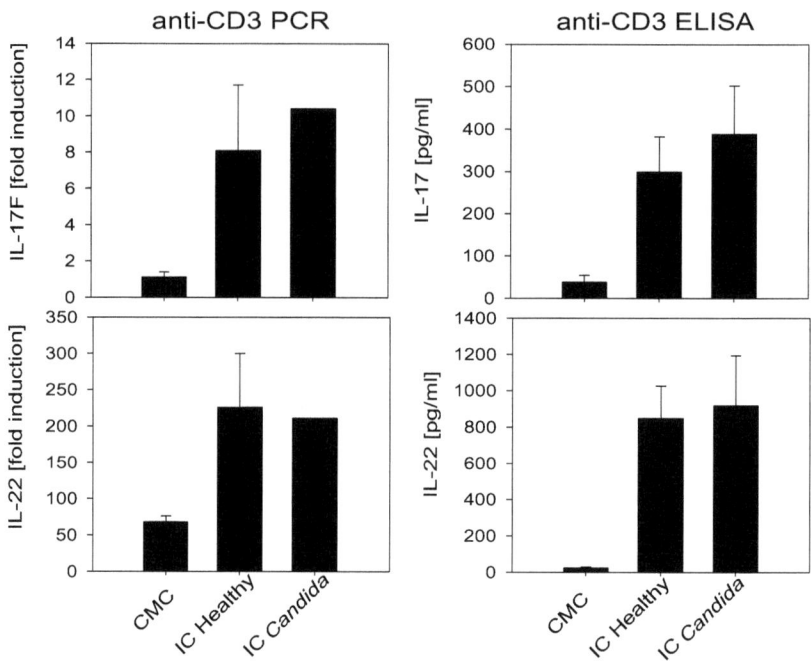

*Figure 10. Directly stimulated T cells of CMC patients secrete diminished levels of IL-17 and IL-22. Secretion of IL-17 (upper panel) and IL-22 (lower panel) is given at the y-axis. Shown is the mean of three independent experiments (3 CMC patients, 8 healthy controls, 2 Candidiasis patients in total). Error bars indicate mean +/- SEM. (CMC: chronic mucocutaneous candidasis; IC healthy: immune competent volunteers; IC Candida: immune competent Candidiasis patients)*

To investigate the main source of IL-17 within the T cell compartment, we isolated purified CD4+ and CD8+ T cells and co-cultured them with autologous monocytes as antigen-presenting cells and *Candida albicans*. These experiments revealed that IL-17 and IL-22 are predominantly derived from CD4+ T cells. In contrast, only a very low amount of IL-17 and IL-22 was secreted by the CD8+ T cell compartment. Thus, the disability of CMC patients to produce IL-17 and IL-22 is mainly attributed to CD4+ T cells (Figure 11).

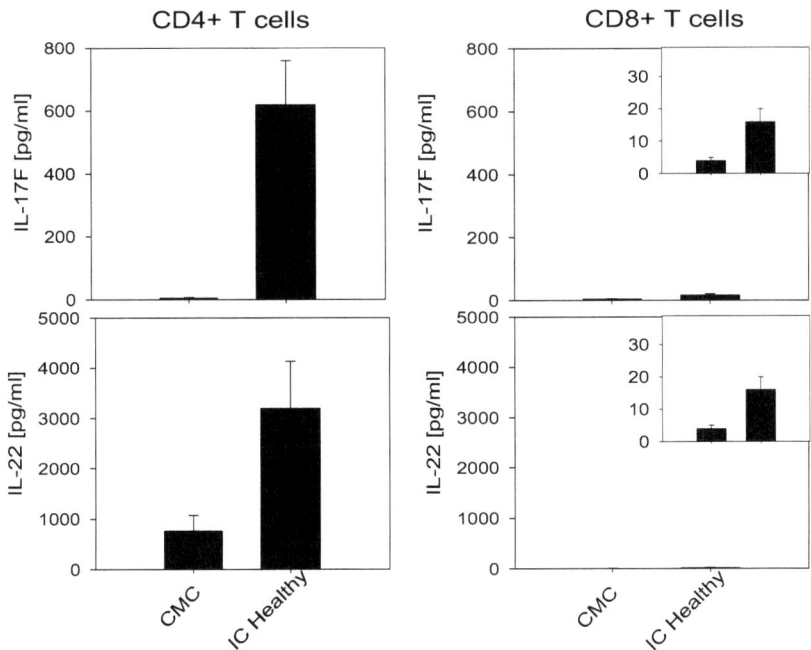

*Figure 11. CD4+ T helper cells are the main source of IL-17 and IL-22. Secretion of IL-17 (upper panel) and IL-22 (lower panel) of CD4+ (left panel) and CD8+ (right panel) T cells is given at the y-axis. The inset in the right panel shows cytokine secretion in pg/ml in a lower scale. Shown is the mean of three independent experiments (2 CMC patients and 5 healthy controls in total). Error bars indicate mean +/- SEM. (CMC: chronic mucocutaneous candidasis; IC healthy: immune competent volunteers)*

*CMC patients exhibit reduced total number of IL-17 producing T cells but normal amounts of CCR4+/CCR6+ T cells*

To answer the question whether CMC patients lack Th17 cells, we quantified IL-17 producing T cells in CMC patients and healthy volunteers. Since CCR4 and CCR6 are described to be good markers for Th17 cells *in vitro*, we first stained PBMC of CMC patients and healthy controls for CCR4 and CCR6 (Figure 12).

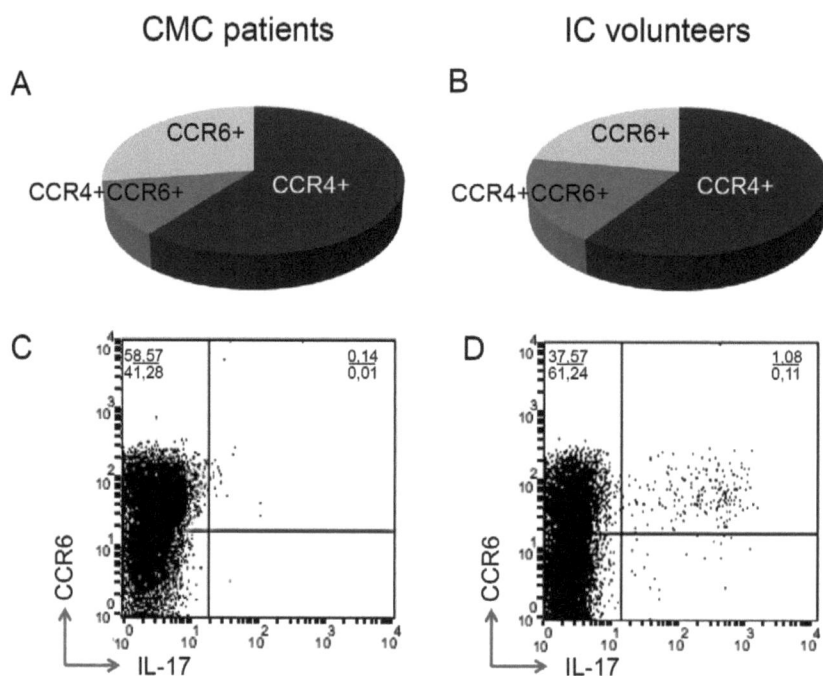

*Figure 12: The CCR6+ IL-17A+ cell population is strongly decreased in CMC patients, while the number of CCR4+CCR6+ cells is not diminished. PBMC of CMC patients and healthy controls were stained intracellularly after PMA/ionomycine stimulation for IL-17 (C,D) (one representative experiment of 3 performed is shown) and analysed for the expression of the surface markers CCR4 and CCR6 (A,B) by flow cytometry (CMC patients n=3 and healthy controls n=4).*

We observed no differences in the relative frequency of CCR4+, CCR6+ or double positive T cells on total PBMC (Figure 12A,B) between CMC and immune competent controls.

However, CCR4+CCR6+ T cells from CMC patients did not produce any IL-17 protein. In contrast, a proportion of CCR6+ cells of healthy controls showed an intracellular accumulation of IL-17 after PMA/ionomycine stimulation (Figure 12C,D). Thus, in line with the secretion profile observed in ELISA, CMC patients show a dramatic decrease of IL-17 producing T cells.

*PBMC of CMC patients are able to secrete Th17-differentiating and -maintaining cytokines*

The absence of IL-17 and IL-22 producing T cells in CMC patients could be the consequence of an impaired differentiation of these cells. Since IL-1β and IL-6 are important for the differentiation of human IL-17 producing T cells, we analysed the expression of IL-1β and IL-6 at the transcriptional level by real time PCR. PBMC of CMC patients stimulated with *Candida albicans* for 12 hours tended to show higher mRNA expression of IL-1β and IL-6 compared to healthy controls (Figure 13). Thus, the observed defect in IL-17 producing T cells in CMC does not involve Th17-differentiating cytokines IL-1β and IL-6.

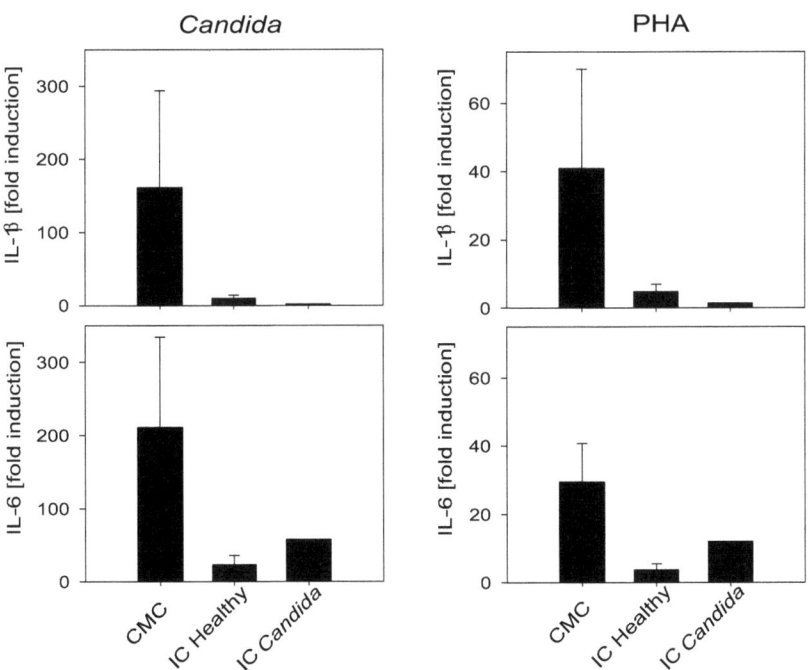

*Figure 13: No significant differences in induction of Th17-differentiating cytokines between CMC patients and immune competent controls. Induction of IL-1β (upper panel) and IL-6 (lower panel) mRNA is given at the y-axis. Shown is the mean of*

*three independent experiments (3 CMC patients, 4 healthy controls, 1 Candidiasis patient in total). Error bars indicate mean +/- SEM.*

## 4.2 IL-17 is involved in a pro-inflammatory *circulus vitiosus* in atopic eczema

*IL-17 producing T lymphocytes are infiltrating the skin during an APT reaction: newly characterised Th2/IL-17 subset*

AE patients characteristically suffer from chronic skin colonisation with *Staphylococcus aureus*, and the density of colonisation directly correlates with disease severity. Since we observed in the first part of this study that the lack of IL-17 and IL-22 results in chronic skin infections (like in CMC patients), we investigated whether also PBMC from AE patients might show a defect in the production of IL-17 and IL-22. For that purpose, three AE patients with documented type I hypersensitivity to *Dermatophagoides pteronyssinus* (Der p) were challenged with Atopy Patch Tests (APT) of Der p. Biopsies were taken from the resulting eczematous reactions and infiltrating T cells were isolated and characterised by intracellular cytokine staining using flow cytometry techniques. In line with the hypothesis of a Th2 domination in early AE, the majority of skin derived T cells activated *in vitro* by PMA plus ionomycine expressed high levels of IL-4 (Figure 14). Moreover, about 9% (9% +/- 3%) of all infiltrated T cells were capable of producing IL-17. IL-17 and IL-22 were not necessarily co-expressed (Figure 14). Interestingly, about one third of IL-17 releasing T cells co-expressed IL-4 (Th2/IL-17 T cells) or IL-4 plus IFN-$\gamma$ (Th0/IL-17 T cells). 50% of IL-17 producing T cells were pure Th17 T cells, a minor proportion coproduced IL-17 and IFN-$\gamma$ (Th1/IL-17) (Figure 14).

*A subpopulation of Der p 1 specific T cells has the capacity to produce IL-17*

In order to further characterise skin-derived IL-17 producing T lymphocytes, T cell lines isolated from biopsied positive APT reactions to Der p were cloned by limiting dilution. Expanded T cell clones (in total 142 T cell clones obtained from 3 AE patients) were characterized for Der p 1 specificity, chemokine receptor expression, as well as the release of IFN-$\gamma$, IL-4, IL-10, IL-13, IL-17, IL-22 and TNF-$\alpha$.

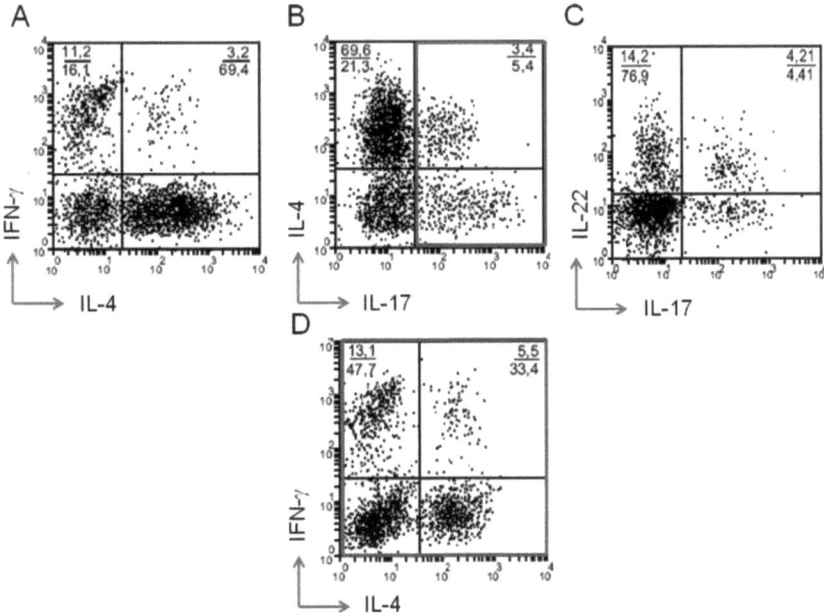

*Figure 14: Distinct populations of IL-17 producing T cells in the skin infiltrate of a positive APT reaction. A: Intracellular cytokine staining of skin-derived lymphocytes with IL-4/IFN-γ (left dot plot), IL-4/IL-17 (middle dot plot) and IL-17/IL-22 (right dot plot). Gating on IL-17+ cells after triple staining with IL-4, IFN-γ and IL-17 (dot plot lower panel). Percentage of cells is indicated for each quadrant. Shown is one representative experiment.*

Consistent with the observations obtained from the APT derived T cell line, a high number of APT derived T cells (24% +/- 1,9%) was capable of producing IL-17 after activation with PMA plus ionomycine. The newly identified subset Th2/IL-17 was identified also on clonal level. The relative distribution of IL-17 producing subpopulations was comparable to the results obtained from T cell lines (Figure 15), with more than 40% pure Th17 phenotype (41% +/- 4,1%), one third Th2/IL-17 (32% +/- 3,6%) and one fourth Th1/IL-17 cells (26% +/- 4,5%). Representative intracellular cytokine stainings for each IL-17 producing subtype are shown in figure 16.

Pure Th17 cells were not specific for Der p 1. Likewise the skin-derived T cell lines, a correlation of IL-17 with IL-22 was not obvious on clonal level. 69% (+/- 4,8%) of skin infiltrating T cell clones were capable of producing IL-22 (Figure 15, Table in the appendix). A characterisation of IL-17 producing T cell clones is shown in table 9 and table 10.

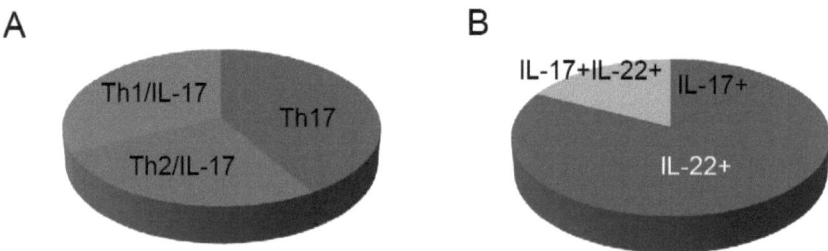

*Figure 15. Cytokine production of T cell clones. A: relative distribution of pure Th17, Th1/IL-17 and Th2/IL-17 clones on total IL-17+ clones. B: percentage of IL-17 secreting, IL-22 secreting and double secreting T cell clones.*

| Clone | Proliferation | | Cytokine Profile (after PMA/ionomycine stimulation) | | | | | | | Subtype |
|---|---|---|---|---|---|---|---|---|---|---|
| | SI to Der p 1 | SI to SEB | IFN-γ | IL-4 | IL-10 | IL-13 | IL-17 | IL-22 | TNF-α | |
| 3 | 75 | 45 | 496 | 4285 | 13484 | 13738 | 12494 | 2931 | 7779 | Th2/IL-17 |
| 27 | 1 | 20 | 0 | 3 | 1578 | 947 | 13788 | 2595 | 1596 | Th17 |
| 60 | 25 | 30 | 5385 | 2922 | 10623 | 13074 | 11000 | 126 | 5348 | Th0/IL-17 |
| 91 | 20 | 15 | 0 | 3252 | 16260 | 18317 | 3519 | 7000 | 4620 | Th2/IL-17 |
| 96 | 40 | 45 | 9946 | 3477 | 16159 | 14302 | 2394 | 3568 | 3840 | Th0/IL-17 |
| 141 | 40 | 1 | 0 | 4710 | 1149 | 20472 | 5500 | 219 | 861 | Th2/IL-17 |

*Table 9. Der p 1 specificity and cytokine secretion profile of IL-17 producing T cell clones obtained from AE patients.*

| Clone | TCR Vβ chain | Surface markers (in resting state) | | | | |
|---|---|---|---|---|---|---|
| | | CD4 | CD8 | CCR4 | CCR6 | CXCR3 |
| 3 | 14 | 94% | 0% | 73% | 85% | 14% |
| 27 | 12 | 98% | 0% | 95% | 99% | 1% |
| 60 | 3 | 96% | 2% | 85% | 90% | 67% |
| 91 | 14 | 98% | 0% | 89% | 50% | 3% |
| 96 | n. det. | 90% | 0% | 1% | 54% | 45% |
| 141 | n. det. | 99% | 0% | 45% | 55% | 1% |

Table 10. TCR analysis and expression of surface markers of IL-17 producing T cell clones obtained from AE patients. Shown is the percentage of positive cells on total cells as compared to isotype control. "n. det." = clone expresses a T cell receptor Vβ chain that is not detectable by the Iotest Beta Mark Repertoire Kit.

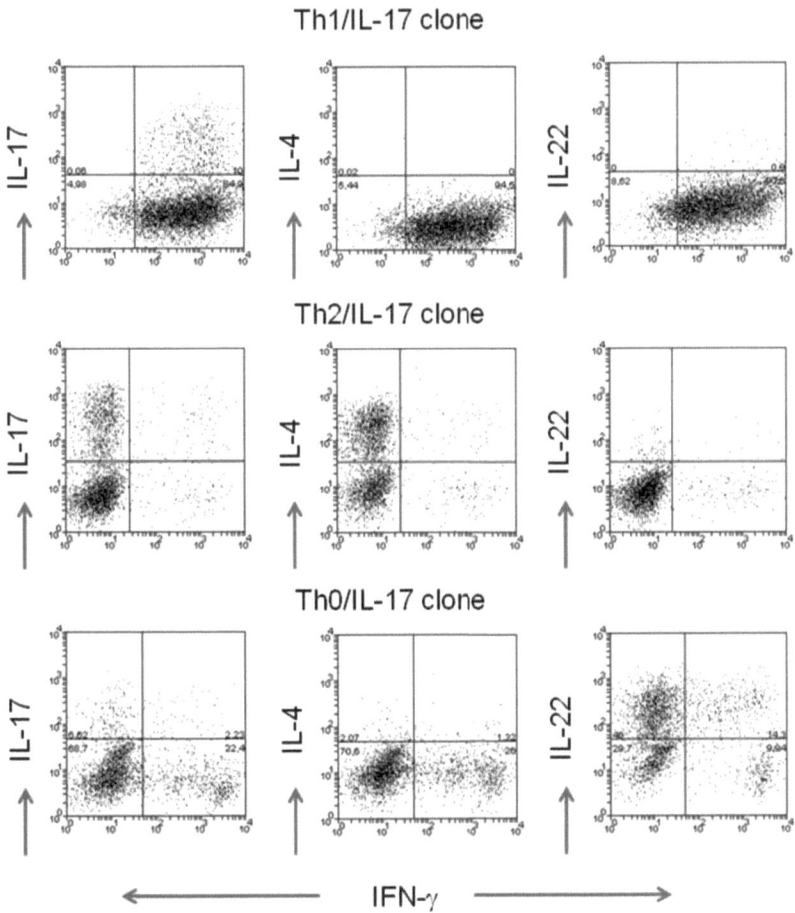

*Figure 16. Intracellular cytokine staining after PMA/ionomycin stimulation of a representative Th1/IL-17, Th2/IL-17 and Th0/IL-17 clone.*

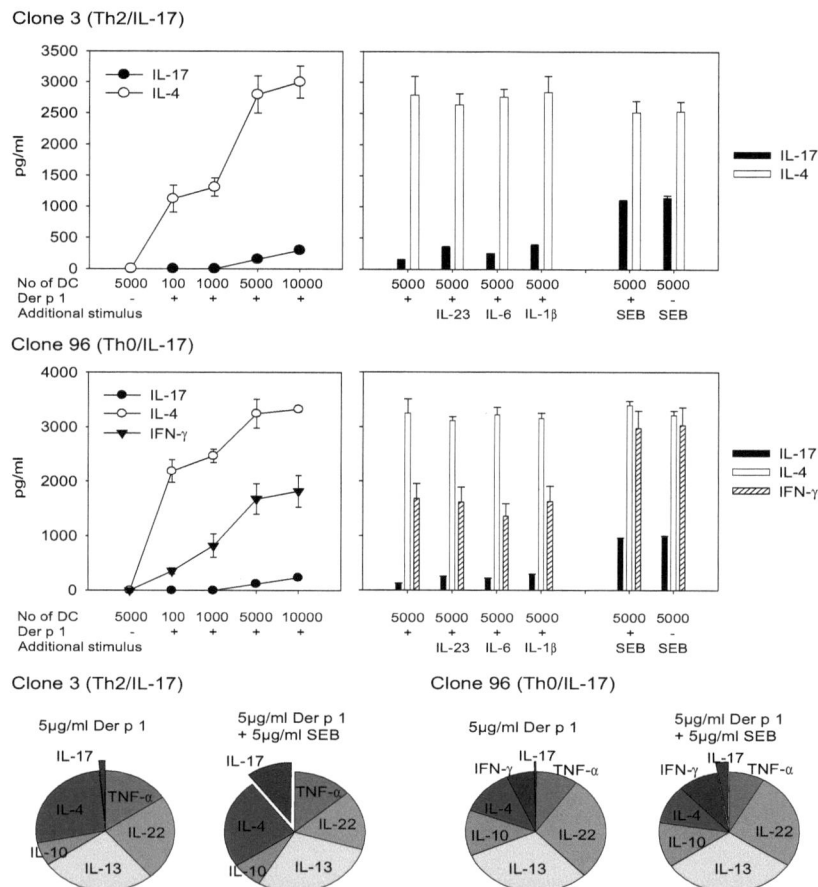

*Figure 17. IL-17+ Der p 1-specific T cell clones secrete IL-17 upon stimulation with SEB, but not with Der p 1. Dose-dependent secretion of IL-17/IL-4/IFN-γ, addition of cytokines and SEB (upper panel). Type of APC: immature DC. Error bars indicate SD of one representative experiment performed in triplicates. Relative cytokine profile (mean % of three independent experiments) of clones is shifted towards IL-17 after stimulation with SEB (lower panel).*

*Stimulation with cognate antigen induces IL-4 and/or IFN-γ release, but no or very low amounts of IL-17*

We then analysed the physiologic reaction pattern of specific skin-derived Th2/IL-17 and Th0/IL-17 T cell clones stimulated with native or recombinant Der p 1 in the presence of different antigen presenting cells (APC). Surprisingly, IL-17 was not or only marginally secreted by Der p 1-specific Th2/IL-17 and Th0/IL-17 cells when the allergen was presented by varying numbers of immature DC (Figure 17). This picture did not change when we co-cultured T cell clones with mature DC (Figure 18) or CD14+ monocytes (Figure 19).

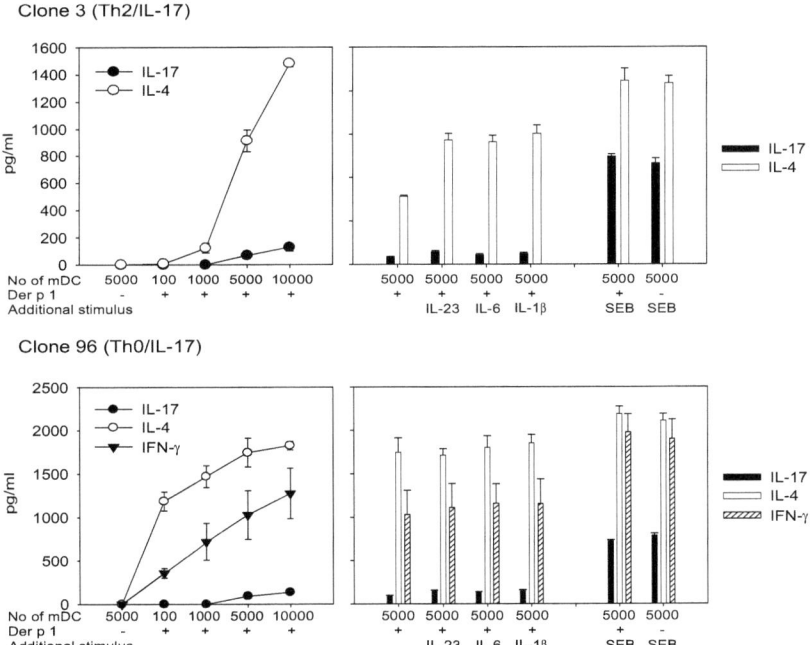

*Figure 18. IL-17+ Der p 1-specific T cell clones secrete IL-17 upon stimulation with SEB, but not with Der p 1. Dose-dependent secretion of IL-17/IL-4/IFN-γ, addition of cytokines and SEB (upper panel). Type of APC: mature DC. Error bars indicate SD of one representative experiment performed in triplicates.*

Increasing the T cell receptor stimulation intensity by stimulation with higher allergen concentration (Figure 20) or the number of APC only marginally upregulated IL-17 secretion (Figures 17-19). In contrast, even at low levels of stimulation intensity (DC: T cell ratio 1:1000 and 5µg/ml Der p 1), high amounts of IL-4 and a strong induction of proliferation were detected, without substantial differences between different APC populations. Thus, in contrast to the maximal stimulation induced by PMA and ionomycin, physiological TCR triggering failed to upregulate the release of IL-17, albeit capable of inducing Th2 cytokines which predominate the early phase of AE.

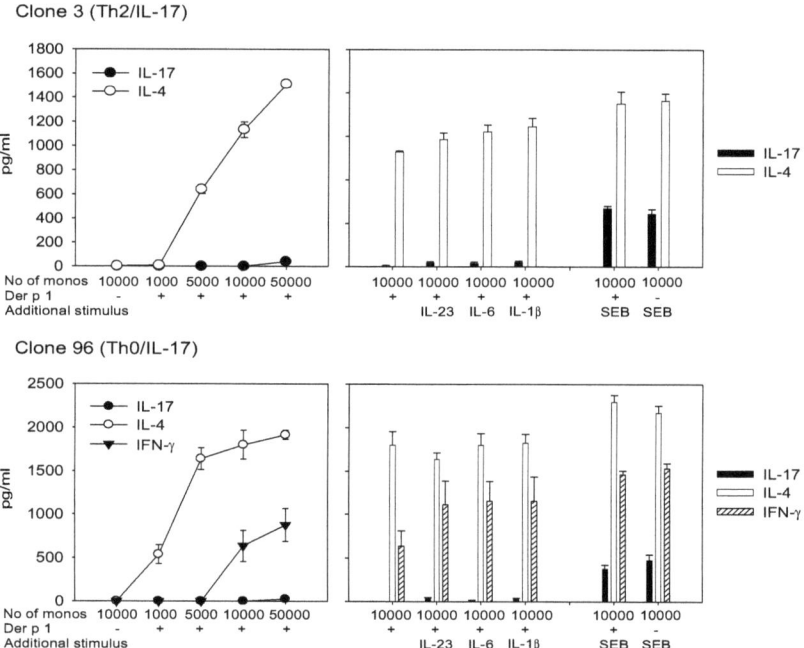

Figure 19. IL-17+ Der p 1-specific T cell clones secrete IL-17 upon stimulation with SEB, but not with Der p 1. Dose-dependent secretion of IL-17/IL-4/IFN-γ, addition of cytokines and SEB (upper panel). Type of APC: monocytes. Error bars indicate SD of one representative experiment performed in triplicates.

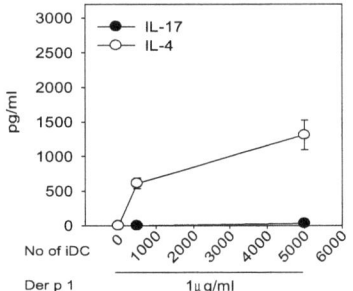 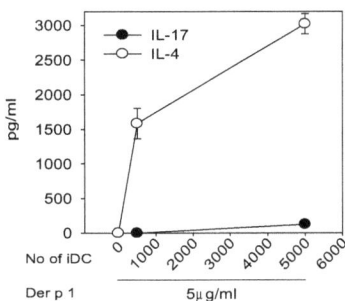

*Figure 20. IL-4 secretion of Der p 1 specific Th2/IL-17 clone is dependent on allergen dose, but IL-17 secretion is not. Shown is the cytokine production of clo ne 3 (Th2/IL-17) after stimulation with increasing amounts of immature DC (x-axis) and the cognate allergen Der p 1 (panels). Error bars indicate standard error of the mean.*

*Th17 associated cytokines IL-1β, IL-6 and IL-23 do not increase IL-17 secretion in allergen-specific stimulated effector T cell clones*

To explain the divergence between the capacity of T cell clones to produce IL-17 and the *de facto* secretion upon cognate antigen recognition, we tried to identify tissue-derived stimuli that could induce IL-17 secretion in Th2/IL-17 and Th0/IL-17 cells. In a first step, we investigated the effect of so far identified cytokines known to be involved in differentiation and maintenance of human Th17 cells. Neither addition of IL-1β, IL-6 nor IL-23 increased IL-17 secretion after stimulation with DC and Der p 1 (Figures 17-19), thus these cytokines seem unlikely to play a role in cytokine secretion of differentiated effector T cells.

*Staphylococcal enterotoxin B induces high secretion of IL-17 by Der p 1-specific T cells*

Since a defect in IL-17 secretion results in recurrent infections of skin and mucosal membranes (chronic mucocutaneous candidiasis, see 4.1), we investigated if microbial derived products could induce substantial production of IL-17. We stimulated skin-derived Der p 1 specific T cell clones (n=5) with the proinflammatory bacterial substances LPS and SEB, which is commonly present on AE skin. While

50μg/ml LPS did not alter the cytokine secretion of T cell clones, addition of 5μg/ml SEB to DC-T cell co-culture strongly promoted IL-17 release by T cells expressing SEB-sensitive TCR Vβ chains (four out of five), (Figures 17-19).

Secretion of IL-10 and of IFN-γ, but not that of IL-4, was also affected in these clones. However, increase of IL-17 secretion was by far most prominent, resulting in an increased percentage relative to other T cell cytokines in all clones examined (Figure 17 lower panel). A predominating Vβ chain was not detected in IL-17 producing T cell clones (Table 10). In line with the literature, blocking TCR by adding neutralizing antibodies against MHC class II molecules abrogated SEB stimulation almost completely (Figure 21). This finding indicates that secretion of inflammatory IL-17 by T lymphocytes is tightly regulated, and requires additional stimulation beyond cognate antigen presentation by professional APC. In AE, such hyper-stimulation could be provided by microbial-derived superantigens.

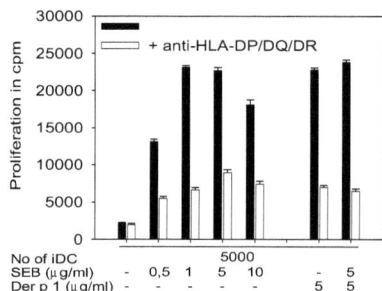 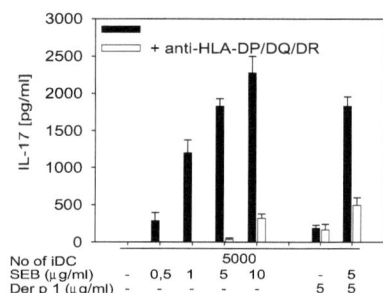

Figure 21. SEB activates T cells through a TCR dependent mechanism. Clone 3 was stimulated with increasing amounts of SEB and immature DC. Experimental endpoints were proliferation (left panel) and IL-17 secretion (right panel). Addition of anti-HLA-DP/DQ/DR almost completely abrogated SEB stimulation (white bars). Error bars indicate SEM of two independent experiments.

*IL-17 strongly induces HBD-2 in vitro, but this effect is diminished in AE.*

To clarify whether the ineffective upregulation of antimicrobial peptides by keratinocytes in AE is due to intrinsic defects in AE keratinocytes or due to inhibitory effects of the microenvironment, we stimulated primary keratinocytes from AE patients (n=3) and healthy donors (n=3) with different T cell cytokines. We found that IL-17 strongly induced HBD-2 release in both AE and healthy keratinocytes *in vitro* (Figure 22). However, IL-17-induced HBD-2 upregulation was partially inhibited by addition of the Th2 cytokines IL-4 and IL-13. Accordingly, experiments performed with supernatants from APT-derived T cell clones demonstrated that neither Th2 nor Th0 could induce HBD-2 release by AE keratinocytes. Th17-derived supernatant was the most effective in HBD-2 induction, whereas the co-expression of IL-4 in the supernatant of Th2/IL-17 partially, but not completely, blocked the induction of HBD-2 release. Finally, pre-incubation of Th17 and Th2/IL-17 supernatant with a neutralizing antibody against IL-17 abrogated HBD-2 induction almost completely (Figure 22).

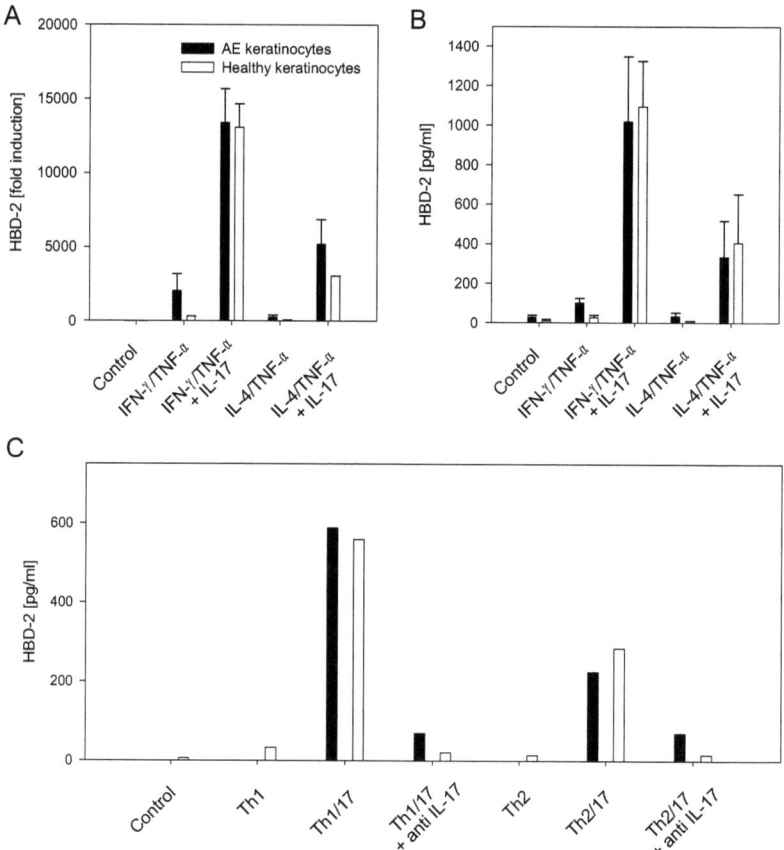

*Figure 22. T cell-derived IL-17 induces β-defensin2 in primary human keratinocytes, IL-4 and IL-13 partially block this effect. Induction of HBD-2 mRNA (left panel) and protein (middle) in AE and healthy keratinocytes in response to recombinant cytokines and to cell-free supernatant obtained from stimulated T cell clones (right panel). Error bars indicate SEM of three independent experiments.*

These data indicate that keratinocytes from AE patients are not hypo-responsive to IL-17, but rather the Th2-dominated microenvironment impairs important effector functions of IL-17.

*SEB strongly upregulates HBD-2 mRNA and protein release in Der p-induced atopic eczema in vivo*

To confirm the role of superantigens in triggering the IL-17/HBD-2 axis *in vivo*, we applied Der p on the two forearms of an AE patient. 36 hours after allergen application, we added 50μg/cm² SEB on one forearm. In concordance with previous reportscxxvii, the clinical reaction was severely aggravated (classified as "+++++" vs. "+++" according to the European Task Force on Atopic Dermatitis [ETFAD] 2000 reading keycxxx) and maintained substantially longer (10 days vs. 4 days) in the SEB-exposed lesion. Sixty hours after allergen application, epidermal sheets of induced eczematous reactions were obtained by the method of suction blister and suction blister fluid was investigated for cytokine content.

In line with our *in vitro* results, IL-17 was induced more than two fold in the SEB challenged Patch Test site, while IFN-γ was unchanged. IL-4 was below detection level, and IL-10 was marginally increased (Figure 23). Consequently, HBD-2 mRNA was two fold increased in keratinocytes from SEB-exposed epidermal sheets. Increased HBD-2 concentration in the SEB-treated APT reaction was confirmed at protein level by ELISA assays performed on the blister fluids (Figure 23).

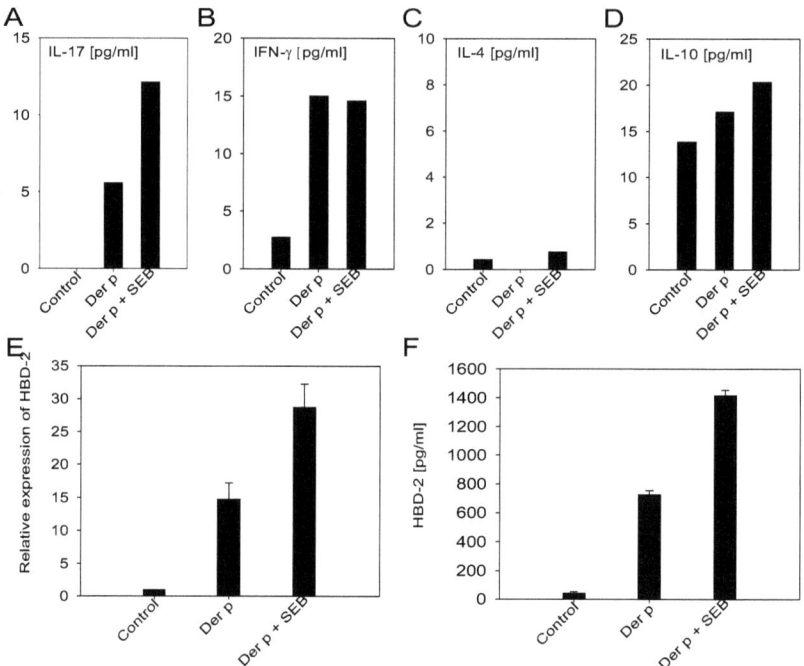

Figure 23. SEB induces expression of IL-17 and HBD-2 in vivo. Levels of IL-17 (A), IFN-γ (B), IL-4 (C) and IL-10 (D) in suction blister fluids as detected by Luminex analysis. E: relative induction of HBD-2 mRNA (E) and protein content (F). Error bars indicate SD of one experiment performed in triplicates.

These data indicate that microbial-derived products might play an essential role in inducing IL-17 *in vivo*.

## 5 Discussion

This work highlights an essential role for IL-17 in the first-line defence of barrier organs. It illustrates that loss of IL-17 results in chronic infections limited to skin and mucosal membranes, which is the underlying pathogenesis of the orphan human disease "chronic mucocutaneous candidiasis". Mechanisms by which IL-17 acts are characterised in the second part of this manuscript, the description of the role of IL-17 in atopic eczema. It reveals that IL-17 is important in coordinating an effective immune response by instructing epithelial cells to an innate immune response and by recruiting immune cells to the site of infection; in atopic eczema, however, such effects are outbalanced by inhibiting effects of the Th2-dominated microenvironment, which results again in chronic infections of the skin.

### 5.1 CMC patients suffer from an impaired Th17 immune response

Patients suffering from CMC show a characteristic pattern of infection with the yeast Candida: while skin and mucosal membranes are heavily attacked, no systemic *Candida* infections are reported. Recent data suggest that the inability to clear *Candida albicans* in CMC patients is based upon a complex heterogeneity of immune defect(s), probably characteristic for various disease subgroups. In the first part of this thesis, a main pathogenic mechanism of CMC is elucidated – a deficiency in the production of the Th17-associated cytokines IL-17 and IL-22. Interestingly, mediators important for differentiation (IL-6 and IL-1β) and maintenance (IL-23) of the Th17 lineage were enhanced or not altered.

*The role of Th17 cells in* Candida *infections*
First evidence for the importance of IL-17 in clearing *Candida* infections has been provided in the mouse system: IL-17A receptor knockout mice showed a dose-dependent, substantially reduced survival in a murine model of systemic candidiasis[xxxii] . Recent data revealed that infection with *Candida albicans* leads to an induction of murine IL-17 producing T cells[cxxx]. Furthermore, the hyphal form of

*Candida albicans* triggers IL-17 production of freshly isolated human CD4+ T cells of healthy donors *in* vitro[xxxiv].

An important role for IL-17 producing T cells in clearing *Candida* infections is confirmed by results demonstrated in this work, as PBMC of immune competent patients suffering from *Candida* infections showed a significantly higher secretion of IL-17 and IL-22 after *in vitro* stimulation with *Candida albicans* compared to healthy (non-Candida infected) donors. In concordance with previous reports[xxviii,cxxxi,cxliii], the source of IL-17 in PBMC was almost exclusively limited to CD4+ CCR-6+ T cells. T cell receptor specific stimulation of PBMC and stimulation of isolated CD4+ T cells with autologous monocytes showed comparable amounts of secreted IL-17, indicating that IL-17 was predominantly derived from CD4+ T cells. Flow cytometry analysis of PBMC revealed nearly all cells positive for IL-17 in intracellular staining were also CCR-6 positive.

## CMC patients suffer from an impaired Th17 immune response

However, even though they had been chronically exposed to *Candida albicans*, PBMC from CMC patients secreted significantly lower amounts of IL-17 and IL-22 than PBMC from healthy donors and patients with current *Candida* infection after stimulation with *Candida albicans in vitro* - both on the mRNA and on protein level. The underlying immune defect was not specific for the stimulus *Candida*, as mitogen stimulation (PHA) and T cell receptor specific stimulation (anti-CD3/anti-CD28) also resulted in a reduced secretion of IL-17 and IL-22 in CMC patients. This decrease was due to a strongly diminished total number of IL-17 producing T cells, as detected by surface CCR-6 and intracellular IL-17 staining of PBMC by flow cytometry. The weaker secretion of IL-22 was less pronounced than that of IL-17 as compared to immune competent patients either infected or non-infected with *Candida*. This could be explained by the fact that IL-22 production is not limited to Th17 cells, but is also produced by other activated T cell subtypes[xxxv,cxxxii].

## Th17-differentiating cytokines are not diminished in CMC patients

The so far identified differentiation factors for human IL-17 producing T cells are IL-1β and IL-6[xxii], whereas IL-23 seems to be important for maintaining the production of IL-17 and IL-22 in mouse[cxxxiii,cxxxiv,cxliv], but to a lesser degree in human IL-17 producing T cells[xxii] (see 1.1). IL-21 and TGF-β are important differentiation factors in the mouse, but their role is still controversial in humans. While IL-21 does not seem to play a role in the human system[cxxxv], the role of TGF-β is still under debate with some authors arguing it is not required for differentiation[xxii] and others observing a dependence of Th17 differentiation on presence of TGF-β[ξξιϖ]. To investigate if CMC patients lack one of these Th17-associated cytokines, we measured the induction of IL-1β, IL-6 and IL-23 after stimulation of PBMC with both specific and mitogenic stimuli. We observed a strong enhancement of IL-1β and IL-6, but not of IL-23. The secretion of these cytokines in PBMC of patients suffering from CMC was not diminished. In contrast, mRNA expression of IL-1β and IL-6 was induced much stronger in CMC patients, resulting in slightly higher release of proteins after 72 hours. This could indicate a defect in differentiation or survival of IL-17 producing T cells downstream of IL-1β and IL-6.

*Mechanisms of candidicidal activity of IL-17*
Concerning the mechanism of the candidicidal effects of IL-17 producing T cells, two possible pathways could be involved in clearing infection: there is, on the one hand, the strong neutrophil recruiting capacity of IL-17 via the induction of IL-8 in human keratinocytes[xxxvi]. On the other hand, IL-17 and IL-22 synergistically induce β-defensins in human keratinocytes[xxxviii] that are able to kill *Candida albicans*[cxxxvi,cxxxvii]. More than the described strongly decreased levels of the tissue-instructing cytokines IL-17, IL-22, and IFN-γ, type-2 cytokines such as IL-4 and IL-10 are over-expressed in PBMC of CMC patients[lxxvii]. Importantly, these cytokines further promote an infection of epithelium with *Candida* by counteracting the effects of IL-17[cxxxviii,cxxxix] regarding the induction of antimicrobial peptides (see 4.2) and failed recruitment of phagocytic cells like neutrophil granulocytes by epithelial cells (Figure 24). Taken together, a decrease in the absolute number of IL-17 producing T cells and the resulting diminished stimulation of epithelial cells[cxl] could explain why Candidiasis is limited to skin and mucosal membranes in CMC patients – and help to understand why they do not suffer from a systemic Candidiasis.

In summary this study underlines the importance of IL-17 producing T cells for the clearance of *Candida* infections. Furthermore our data suggest that an impaired IL-17 and IL-22 response seems to be at least in part responsible for the pathogenesis of

CMC. The hypothesis that a failed immune response of "tissue-signaling leukocytes" like Th17 cells leads to chronic infections limited to skin and mucosal membranes is strengthened by a recent report on an impaired Th17 immune response in autosomal-dominant hyper-IgE syndrome – a second orphan disease regularly associated with *Candida* infections limited to skin and mucosa[cxli].

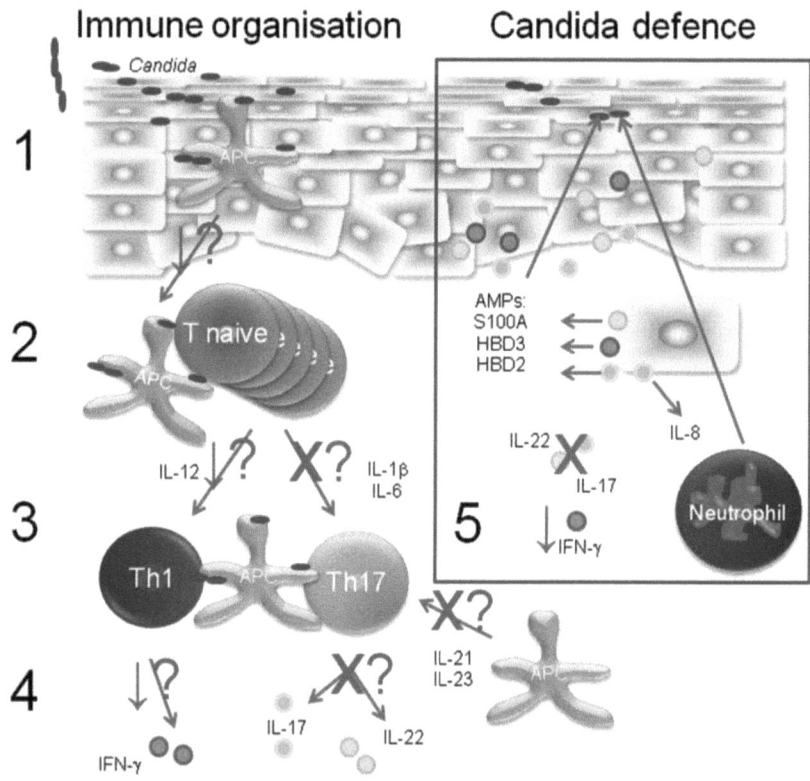

Figure 24. The pathogenesis of CMC. Upon encounter of Candida, antigen presenting cells take up and process antigens (1), then migrate to regional lymph nodes and present them to specific naive T cells (2), which undergo clonal expansion and differentiation towards memory effector cells mainly of the Th1 or Th17 phenotype (3). A second stimulation of T cells with Candida leads to secretion of IFN-γ or IL-17 and IL-22, respectively (4). These cytokines induce secretion of antimicrobial peptides (AMPs) and neutrophil-recruiting IL-8 in epithelial cells (5).

*Lack of IL-17 and IL-22 and diminished IFN-γ results in CMC. The potential defects in this cascade underlying CMC are marked with red "X" or "↓".*

## 5.2 The IL-17 mediated host defence is partially impaired in AE patients

Our results on the pathogenesis of "chronic mucocutaneous candidiasis" suggest a central role of IL-17 in encompassing host defence against microorganisms at surface barriers. This led us to investigate the role of IL-17 in atopic eczema (AE), since almost all AE patients suffer from a chronic skin-colonisation with the bacterium *Staphyloccocus aureus*. Furthermore, disease severity in AE positively correlates with the densitiy of *Staphylococcus aureus* on the skin. This observation led us to investigate IL-17 in the pathogenesis of AE.

*IL-17 producing T cell populations infiltrating AE lesions*
In a first step, we demonstrate that distinct subpopulations of IL-17 secreting T cells infiltrate acute skin lesions, where they trigger keratinocytes to produce the antimicrobial peptide HBD-2. However, this induction is substantially impaired in the presence of type-2 cytokines abundantly present in AE skin microenvironment.
By isolating and characterising the lymphocytic infiltrate in APT reactions, we directly demonstrate IL-17-releasing T cells in acute AE lesions. Hereby we confirm and extend a previous report describing the detection of IL-17 mRNA by PCR in AE skin[cxlii]. When we further characterised skin infiltrating T cells, we identified distinct subpopulations of IL-17 producing T cell clones: besides the previously published pure Th17 and Th1/IL-17 cells that co-express IFN-$\gamma\xi\xi\xi\omega\iota$[cxliii], a newly described population coproducing IL-17 and type 2 cytokines was classified as Th2/IL-17.

*Secretion of IL-17 in T cells is tightly regulated*
While in the APT lesion no Der p 1 specific Th17 cells were found on clonal level, we were surprised to observe that stimulation of Der p 1 specific Th2/IL-17 and Th0/IL-17 cells with their cognate antigen resulted in a strong induction of proliferation and of IL-4 secretion, but IL-17 was poorly secreted. Neither Th17 differentiating cytokines IL-1$\beta$ and IL-6xxii nor IL-23, described to maintain survival and cytokine secretion of mouse[cxliv], but to a lesser degree also of human Th17 cellsxxii, strongly increased secretion of IL-17 in our differentiated effector T cells stimulated with DC and their cognate antigen.

In order to find an *in vivo* stimulus for substantial IL-17 secretion, we investigated whether microbial derived products could be adequate stimuli. Consensus exists that *Staph. aureus* colonisation of AE skin significantly aggravates intensity and accounts for persistence of eczematous reactions[cxxiv,cxxv], however the mechanisms remain unclear. Under natural exposure conditions, *Staph. aureus* derived superantigens, like SEB, could contribute to the amplification of the inflammatory reaction by stimulating infiltrating T cells bearing particular T cell receptor Vβ chains[cxxv,cxxvi]. Indeed, when we stimulated SEB-sensitive Th2/IL-17 and Th0/IL-17 clones with SEB, secretion of proinflammatory IFN-γ, but especially of IL-17, was strongly enhanced compared to cognate TCR triggering alone both *in vitro* and *in vivo*. Thus, our data underline a role of the microenvironment in triggering full effector functions of tissue-infiltrating T cells.

*The role of the local microenvironment for the induction of HBD-2 in keratinocytes*
However, despite availability of SEB-triggered IL-17, which is a very efficient stimulus for HBD-2[xxxviii], expression of HBD-2 in AE was reported to be diminished in comparison to Th1-mediated skin immune diseases, such as psoriasis[cxxiii]. We therefore investigated whether AE keratinocytes show an intrinsic defect in responding to IL-17 or whether co-expressed type 2 cytokines could account for the diminished HBD-2 induction, as reported for the IFN-γ and TNF-α induced expression of antimicrobial peptides[cxlv,cxlvi]. We found that AE keratinocytes are not hypo-responsive to IL-17 *in vitro*, but rather the AE skin microenvironment containing abundant IL-4 and IL-13 partially inhibits the IL-17/HBD-2 axis. This could, at least in part, explain the persistent colonisation of AE skin with *Staph. aureus* that represents a continuous trigger of cutaneous inflammation.

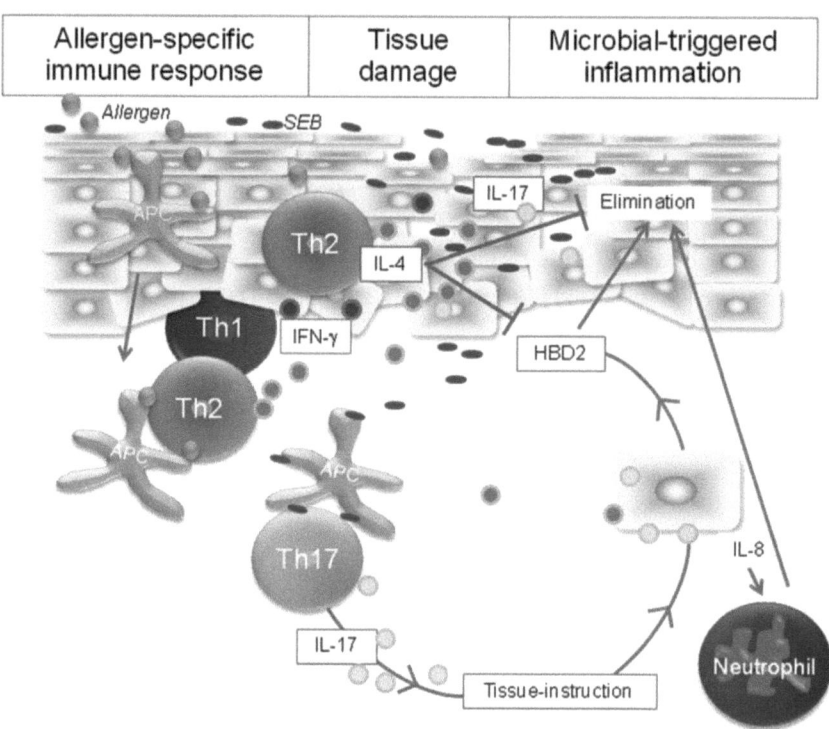

Figure 25. A new concept for the pathogenesis of AE. An initial allergen-specific Th2-dominated immune response causes epidermal barrier disruption and consequent triggering of an IL-17 immune response by microbial-derived substances. IL-17, however, does not signal effectively to epithelial cells due to inhibitory effects of the type 2-dominated microenvironment.

A new concept on the pathogenesis of atopic eczema
Atopic eczema is a common inflammatory skin disorder based upon complex pathogenic mechanisms that altogether result in a disturbed epidermal barrier and cutaneous hyper-inflammation. Our *in vivo* and *in vitro* observations demonstrate that IL-17 is involved in a previously unknown pro-inflammatory *vicious circle* contributing to both epidermal barrier damage and hyper-inflamed skin (Figure 25).

IL-17 producing T cells are recruited into inflamed AE skin, mainly as Th2/IL-17 and Th0/IL-17 subsets. Cognate antigen recognition of causative allergens (e.g. house dust mite) by infiltrating T cells strongly upregulates Th2 cytokines, which dominate the early phase of AE[cxlvii], but only marginally regulates IL-17 secretion. Tissue-derived additional stimuli are required to arm IL-17 releasing T cells. A prerequisite for such a strong stimulation is the loss of the epidermal barrier integrity that builds up the physical and chemical protection against the environment. In the case of AE, the epidermal barrier is altered due to predisposing mutations even in steady state. During an immune reaction in the skin, this barrier is further damaged by two independent cascades: first, the abundantly present type 2 cytokines (IL-4, IL-13) downregulate genes important for building an intact epidermal barrier (e.g. filaggrin)[cxlviii]. Interestingly, filaggrin deficiency in turn promotes a Th17 immune response[cxlix]. Second, the immune reaction in the skin results in keratinocyte apoptosis[cl] and early disruption of E-cadherins[cli]. Both events lead to a complete loss of epidermal integrity and thus to contact of resident and recruited immune cells with microorganisms (*Staph. aureus*) that are colonising the skin of most AE patients.

A second inflammatory wave is now initiated, since *Staph. aureus*-derived superantigens (e.g. SEB) effectively induces IL-17 production in capable T cell clones and thereby initiates the IL-17/HBD-2 axis in the skin. Whereas this mechanism may occur as a natural protective function of IL-17, the IL-17/HBD-2 axis is only marginally effective in AE skin, due to inhibitory effects of Th2 associated cytokines in AE microenvironment[cxlv,cxlvi]. The incomplete clearance of microbial-derived triggers leads to a *vicious circle* responsible for the continuous release of pro-inflammatory IL-17 and other T cell cytokines and persistence of the eczematous reaction.

## 6    Summary

This manuscript demonstrates that IL-17 is crucial in the first-line defence of the human organism by identifying an absent or impaired IL-17 signaling cascade in two human diseases characterised by recurrent infections limited to skin and mucosal membranes.

In the first part we identify the main immune defect in the orphan syndrome "chronic mucocutaneous candidiasis" is an impaired Th17 immune response. CMC patients suffer from a remarkable decrease in IL-17 and IL-22 producing leukocytes, while a specific stimulation with the disease-relevant yeast Candida albicans caused a massive production of IL-17 and IL-22 in healthy volunteers and even more in immune competent Candida-infected patients. The underlying mechanisms remains unknown, a mutation in a Th17-differentiating gene, however, seems unlikely based on the data provided in this thesis. Secondly, we investigated another disease commonly associated with limited skin infections – atopic eczema (AE). Almost 100% of AE patients suffer from a disease-relevant skin colonisation with *Staphylococcus aureus*, most likely due to a diminished production of (IL-17 triggered) defensins. The current study demonstrates that IL-17 producing T cells infiltrate acute AE reactions, in particular the newly characterized subtype Th2/IL-17 cells. Interestingly, T cells challenged with their cognate allergen do not produce IL-17 *in vitro*; but IL-17 secretion can be triggered by *Staphylococcal*-derived enterotoxins (SEB) that are frequently present on AE skin. To analyse why IL-17 can be efficiently triggered in AE, but yet it´s main function (the induction of defensins in keratinocytes) is diminished, primary human keratinocytes from AE patients and healthy volunteers were stimulated with natural and recombinant IL-17. It could be shown that the inefficient defensin induction is not due to an intrinsic defect in AE keratinocytes, but rather due to counteracting effects of Th2 cytokines like IL-4 and IL-13.

This manuscript provides insights in the importance of the skin microenvironment for the outcome of (T cell) mediated immune responses. Furthermore, it is of clinical relevance as 1.) the description of an impaired Th17 immune response in CMC patients could result in specific therapeutic approaches and 2.) it underlines the importance of early and consequent therapy of AE skin lesions to avoid insufficient and persistent triggering of the IL-17/HBD-2 axis in ongoing acute AE.

# 7 References

[i] Von Andrian UH, Mackay CR. T-cell function and migration. Two sides of the same coin. N Engl J Med. 2000; 343: 1020-34.

[ii] Sallusto F, Lanzavecchia A. Heterogeneity of CD4+ memory T cells: functional modules for tailored immunity. Eur J Immunol. 2009; 39: 2076-82.

[iii] Dardalhon V, Awasthi A, Kwon H, Galileos G, Gao W, Sobel RA, Mitsdoerffer M, Strom TB, Elyaman W, Ho IC, Khoury S, Oukka M, Kuchroo VK. IL-4 inhibits TGF-beta-induced Foxp3+ T cells and, together with TGF-beta, generates IL-9+IL-10+Foxp3(-) effector T cells. Nat Immunol. 2008; 9:1347-55.

[iv] Korn T, Bettelli E, Oukka M, Kuchroo VK. IL-17 and Th17 cells. Annu Rev Immunol. 2009; 27: 485-517.

[v] Duhen T, Geiger R, Jarossay D, Lanzavecchia A, Sallusto F. Production of interleukin-22 but not interleukin-17 by a subset of human skin-homing memory T cells. Nat Immunol. 2009; 10: 857-63.

[vi] Trifari S, Kaplan CD, Tran EH, Crellin NK, Spits H. Identification of a human helper T cell population that has abundant production of interleukin 22 and is distinct from T(H)17, T(H)1 and T(H)2 cells. Nat Immunol. 2009; 10: 864-71.

[vii] Eyerich S, Eyerich K, Pennino D, Carbone T, Nasorri F, Pallotta S, Cianferani F, Odorisio T, Traidl-Hoffmann C, Behrendt H, Durham SR, Schmidt-Weber C, Cavani A. Th22 cells represent a distinct human T cell subset involved in epidermal immunity and remodeling. J Clin Invest, In press.

[viii] Liu H, Leung BP. CD4+CD25+ regulatory T cells in health and disease. Clin Exp Pharmacol Physiol. 2006; 33: 519-24.

[ix] Zhou L, Lpes JE, Chong MM, Ivanov II, Min R, Victora GD, Shen Y, Du J, Rubtsov YP, Rudensky AY, Ziegler SF, Littman DR. TGF-beta-induced Foxp3 inhibits T(H)17 cell differentiation by antagonizing RORgammat function. Nature. 2008; 453: 236-40.

[x] Kryczek I, Wei S, Zou L, Altuwaijri S, Szeliga W, Kolls J, Chang A, Zhou W. Cutting edge: T17 and regulatory T cell dynamics and the regulation by IL-2 in the tumor microenvironment. J Immunol. 2007; 178: 6730-3.

[xi] Satoh-Takayama N, Vosshenrich CA, Lesjean-Pottier S, Sawa S, Lochner M, Rattis F, Mention JJ, Thiam K, Cerf-Bensussan N, Mandelboim O, Eberl G, Di Santo JP. Immunity. 2008; 29: 958-70.

[xii] Hall JA, Bouladoux N, Sun CM, Wohlfert EA, Blank RB, Zhu Q, Grigg ME, Berzofsky JA, Belkaid Y. Commensal DNA limits regulatory T cell conversion and is a natural adjuvant of intestinal immune responses. Immunity. 2008; 29: 637-49.

[xiii] Manel N, Unutmaz D, Littman DR. The differentiation of human T(H)-17 cells requires transforming growth factor-beta and induction of the nuclear receptor RORgammat. Nat Immunol. 2008; 9: 641-9.

[xiv] Peng MY, Wang ZH, Yao CY, Jianf LN, Jin QL, Wang J, Li BQ. Interleukin-17-producing gamma delta T cells increased in patients with active pulmonary tuberculosis. Cell Mol Immunol. 2008; 5: 203-8.

[xv] Lockhart E, Green AM, Flynn JL. IL-17 production is dominated by gammadelta T cells rather than CD4 T cells during Mycobacterium tuberculosis infection. J Immunol. 2006; 177: 4662-9.

[xvi] Umemura M, Yahagi A, Hamada S, Begum MD, Watanabe H, Kawakami K, Suda T, Sudo K, Nakae S, Iwakura Y, Matsuzaki G. IL-17-mediated regulation of innate and acquired immune response against pulmonary Mycobacterium bovis bacilli Calmette-Guerin infection. J Immunol. 2007; 178: 3786-96.

[xvii] Hamada S, Umemura M, Shiono T, Tanaka K, Yahagi A, Begum MD, Oshiro K, Okamoto Y, Watanabe H, Kawakami K, Roark C, Born WK, O´Brien R, Ikuta K, Ishiwaka H, Nakae S, Iwakura Y, Ohta T, Matsuzaki G. IL-17A produced by gammadelta T cells play a critical role in innate immunity against listeria monocytogenes infection in the liver. J Immunol. 2008; 181: 3456-63.

[xviii] Roark CL, French JD, Taylor MA, Bendele AM, Born WK, O`Brien RL. Exacerbation of collagen-induced arthritis by oligoclonal, IL-17-producing gamma delta T cells. J Immunol. 2007; 179: 5576-83.

[xix] Romani L, Fallarino F, De Luca A, Montagnoli C, D´Angelo C, Zelante T, Vacca C, Bistoni F, Fioretti MC, Grohmann U, Segal BH, Puccetti P. Defective tryptophan catabolism underlies inflammation in mouse chronic granulomatous disease. Nature. 2008; 451: 211-5.

[xx] Ferretti S, Bonneau O, Dubois GR, Jones CE, Trifilieff A. IL-17, produced by lymphocytes and neutrophils, is necessary for lipopoysaccharide-induced airway neutrophilia: IL-15 as a possible trigger. J Immunol. 2003; 170: 2106-12.

[xxi] Langrish CL, Chen Y, Blumenschein WM, Mattson J, Basham B, Sedgwick JD, McClanahan T, Kastelein RA, Cua DJ. IL-23 drives a pathogenic T cell population that induces autoimmune inflammation. J Exp Med. 2005; 201: 233-40.

[xxii] Acosta-Rodriguez EV, Napolitani G, Lanzavecchia A, Sallusto F. Interleukins 1beta and 6 but not transforming growth factor beta are essential for the differentiation of interleukin 17-producing human t helper cells. Nat Immunol. 2007; 8: 942-9.

[xxiii] Zhou L, Ivanov II, Spolski R, Min R, Shenderov K, Egawa T, Levy DE, Leonard WJ, Littman DR. IL-6 programs T(H)-17 cell differentiation by promoting sequential engagement of the IL-21 and IL-23 pathways. Nat Immunol. 2007; 8: 967-74.

[xxiv] Manel N, Urutmaz D, Littman DR. The differentiation of human T(H)-17 cells requires transforming growth factor-beta and induction of the nuclear receptor RORgammat. Nat Immunol. 2008; 9: 641-9.

[xxv] Bauquet AT, Jin H, Paterson AM, Mitsdoerffer M, Ho IC, Sharpe AH, Kuchroo VK. The costimulatory molecule ICOS regulates the expression of c-Maf and IL-21 in the development of follicular T helper cells and TH-17 cells. Nat Immunol. 2009; 10: 167-75.

[xxvi] Aggarwal S, Ghilardi N, Xie MH, de Sauvage FJ, Gurney AL. Interleukin-23 promotes a distinct CD4 T cell activation state characterized by the production of interleukin-17. J Biol Chem. 2003; 278: 1910-4.

[xxvii] Cua DJ, Sherlock J, Chen Y, Murphy CA, Joyce B, Seymour B, Lucian L, To W, Kwan S, Churakova T, Zurawski S, Wiekowski M, Lira SA, Gorman D, Kastelein RA, Sedgwick JD. Interleukin-23 rather than interleukin-12 is the critical cytokine for autoimmune inflammation of the brain. Nature. 2003; 421: 744-8.

[xxviii] Singh SP, Zhang HH, Foley JF, Hedrick MN, Farber JM (2008). Human T cells that are able to produce IL-17 express the chemokine receptor CCR6. J Immunol 180(1):214-21.

[xxix] Cosmi L, De Palma R, Santarlasci V, Maggi L, Capone M, Frosali F, Rodolico G, Querci V, Abbate G, Angeli R, Berrino L, Fambrini M, Caproni M, Tonelli F, Lazzeri E, Parronchi P, Liotta F, Maggi E, Romagnani S, Annunziato F. Human interleukin 17-producing cells originate from a CD161+CD4+ T cell precursor. J Exp Med. 2008; 205: 1903-16.

[xxx] Kleinschek MA, Boniface K, Sadekova S, Grein J, Murphy EE, Turner SP, Raskin L, Desai B, Faubion WA, de Wall Malefyt R, Pierce RH, McClanahan T, Kastelein RA. J Exp Med. 2009; 206: 525-34.

[xxxi] Bettelli E, Korn T, Oukka M, Kuchroo VK. Induction and effector functions of T(H)17 cells. Nature. 2008; 453: 1051-7.

[xxxii] Huang W, Na L, Fidel PL, Schwarzenberger P. Requirement of interleukin-17A for systemic anti-Candida albicans host defense in mice. J Infect Dis. 2004; 190: 624-31.

[xxxiii] Bettelli E, Oukka M, Kuchroo VK (2007). T(H)-17 cells in the circle of immunity and autoimmunity. *Nat Immunol* 8(4):345-50.

[xxxiv] Acosta-Rodriguez EV, Rivino L, Geginat J, Jarrossay D, Gattorno M, Lanzavecchia A, et al (2007). Surface phenotype and antigenic specificity of human interleukin 17-producing T helper memory cells. *Nat Immunol* 8: 639-46.

[xxxv] Conti HR, Shen F, Nayyar N, Stocum E, Sun JN, Lindemann MJ, Ho AW, Hai JH, Yu JJ, Jung JW, Filler SG, Masso-Welch P, Edgerton M, Gaffen SL. Th17 cells and IL-17 receptor signaling are essential for mucosal host defense against oral cnadidiasis. J Exp Med. 2009; 206: 299-311.

[xxxvi] Albanesi C, Scarponi C, Cavani A, Federici M, Nasorri F, Girolomoni G. Interleukin-17 is produced by both Th1 and Th2 lymphocytes, and modulates interferon-gamma- and interleukin-4-induced activation of human keratinocytes. J Invest Dermatol. 2000; 115: 81-7.

[xxxvii] Nograles KE, Zaba LC, Guttman-Yassky E, Fuentes-Duculan J, Suárez-Farinas M, Cardinale I, Khatcherian A, Gonzalez J, Pierson KC, White TR, Pensabene C, Coats I, Novitskaya I, Lowes MA, Krueger JG. Th17 cytokines interleukin (IL)-17 and IL-22 modulate distinct inflammatory and keratinocyte-response pathways. Br J Dermatol. 2008; 159: 1092-102.

[xxxviii] Liang SC, Tan XY, Luxenberg DP, Karim R, Dunussi-Joannopoulos K, Collins M, et al. Interleukin (IL)-22 and IL-17 are coexpressed by Th17 cells and cooperatively enhance expression of antimicrobial peptides. J Exp Med 2006;203:2271-9.

[xxxix] Midorikawa K, Ouhara K, Komatsuzawa H, Kawai T, Yamada S, Fujiwara T, et al. Staphylococcus aureus susceptibility to innate antimicrobial peptides, ☐-defensins and CAP18, expressed by human keratinocytes. Infect Immunity 2003;71:3730-9.

[xl] Yang D, Chertov O, Bykovskaia SN, Chen Q, Buffo MJ, Shogan J, et al. ☐-defensins: linking innate and adaptive immunity through dendritic and T cell CCR6. Science 1999;286:525-528.

[xli] Lebre, M., A. Van der Aar, L. Van Baarsen, T. Van Capel, J. JSchuitemaker, M.L. Kapsenberg, and E. De Jong, Human Keratinocytes Express Functional Toll-Like Receptor 3, 4, 5, and 9. J Invest Dermatol, 2007. 127: p. 331-341.

[xlii] Schroder, J.M. and J. Harder, Antimicrobial skin peptides and proteins. Cell Mol Life Sci, 2006. 63(4): p. 469-86.

[xliii] Gueniche, A., J. Viac, G. Lizard, M. Charveron, and D. Schmitt, Effect of nickel on the activation state of normal human keratinocytes through interleukin 1 and intercellular adhesion molecule 1 expression. Br J Dermatol, 1994. 131(2): p. 250-6.

[xliv] Albanesi, C., C. Scarponi, S. Sebastiani, A. Cavani, M. Federici, S. Sozzani, and G. Girolomoni, A cytokine-to-chemokine axis between T lymphocytes and keratinocytes can favor Th1 cell accumulation in chronic inflammatory skin diseases. J Leukoc Biol, 2001. 70(4): p. 617-23.

[xlv] Pastore, S., S. Corinti, M. La Placa, B. Didona, and G. Girolomoni, Interferon-gamma promotes exaggerated cytokine production in keratinocytes cultured from patients with atopic dermatitis. J Allergy Clin Immunol, 1998. 101(4 Pt 1): p. 538-44.

[xlvi] Charbonnier, A.S., N. Kohrgruber, E. Kriehuber, G. Stingl, A. Rot, and D. Maurer, Macrophage inflammatory protein 3alpha is involved in the constitutive trafficking of epidermal langerhans cells. J Exp Med, 1999. 190(12): p. 1755-68.

[xlvii] Dilulio, N.A., T. Engeman, D. Armstrong, C. Tannenbaum, T.A. Hamilton, and R.L. Fairchild, Groalpha-mediated recruitment of neutrophils is required for elicitation of contact hypersensitivity. Eur J Immunol, 1999. 29(11): p. 3485-95.

[xlviii] Morales, J., B. Homey, A.P. Vicari, S. Hudak, E. Oldham, J. Hedrick, R. Orozco, N.G. Copeland, N.A. Jenkins, L.M. McEvoy, and A. Zlotnik, CTACK, a skin-associated chemokine that preferentially attracts skin-homing memory T cells. Proc Natl Acad Sci U S A, 1999. 96(25): p. 14470-5.

[xlix] Albanesi, C., C. Scarponi, S. Sebastiani, A. Cavani, M. Federici, O. De Pita, P. Puddu, and G. Girolomoni, IL-4 enhances keratinocyte expression of CXCR3 agonistic chemokines. J Immunol, 2000. 165(3): p. 1395-402.

[l] Sebastiani, S., P. Allavena, C. Albanesi, F. Nasorri, G. Bianchi, C. Traidl, S. Sozzani, G. Girolomoni, and A. Cavani, Chemokine receptor expression and function in CD4+ T lymphocytes with regulatory activity. J Immunol, 2001. 166(2): p. 996-1002.

[li] Budnik, A., M. Grewe, K. Gyufko, and J. Krutmann, Analysis of the production of soluble ICAM-1 molecules by human cells. Exp Hematol, 1996. 24(2): p. 352-9.

[lii] Traidl, C., S. Sebastiani, C. Albanesi, H.F. Merk, P. Puddu, G. Girolomoni, and A. Cavani, Disparate cytotoxic activity of nickel-specific CD8+ and CD4+ T cell subsets against keratinocytes. J Immunol, 2000. 165(6): p. 3058-64.

[liii] Trautmann, A., M. Akdis, D. Kleemann, F. Altznauer, H.U. Simon, T. Graeve, M. Noll, E.B. Brocker, K. Blaser, and C.A. Akdis, T cell-mediated Fas-induced keratinocyte apoptosis plays a key pathogenetic role in eczematous dermatitis. J Clin Invest, 2000. 106(1): p. 25-35.

[liv] Trautmann, A., M. Akdis, K. Blaser, and C.A. Akdis, Role of dysregulated apoptosis in atopic dermatitis. Apoptosis, 2000. 5(5): p. 425-9.

[lv] Muller, G., J. Saloga, T. Germann, I. Bellinghausen, M. Mohamadzadeh, J. Knop, and A.H. Enk, Identification and induction of human keratinocyte-derived IL-12. J Clin Invest, 1994. 94(5): p. 1799-805.

[lvi] Dustin, M.L., K.H. Singer, D.T. Tuck, and T.A. Springer, Adhesion of T lymphoblasts to epidermal keratinocytes is regulated by interferon gamma and is mediated by intercellular

adhesion molecule 1 (ICAM-1). J Exp Med, 1988. 167(4): p. 1323-40.

[lvii] Kirkpatrick CH. Chronic mucocutaneous candidiasis. Pediatr Infect Dis J. 2001; 20; 197-206

[lviii] Thorpe ES, Handley HE. Chronic tetany and chronic mycelial stomatitis in a child aged four and one-half years. AMA Am J Dis Child. 1929; 38: 228-38.

[lix] Craig JM, Schiff LH, Boone JE. Chronic moniliasis associated with Addison´s disease. AMA Am J Dis Child. 1955; 89: 669-84.

[lx] Hung W, Migeon CJ, Parrot RH. A possible autoimmune basis for Addison´s disease in three siblings, one with idiopathic hypoparathyroidism, pernicious anemia and superficial moniliasis. N Eng J Med. 1963: 269: 658-63.

[lxi] Chilgren RA, Quie PG, Meuwissen HJ, Hong R. Chronic mucocutaneous candidiasis, deficiency of delayed hypersensitivity, and selective local antibody defect. Lancet. 1967; 2: 688-93.

[lxii] Collins SM, Dominguez M, Ilmarinen T, et al. Dermatological manifestations of autoimmune polyendocrinopathy-candidiasis-ectodermal dystrophy syndrome. Br J Dermatol 2006;154; 1088-1093.

[lxiii] Peterson P, Nagamine K, Scott H, et al. APECED: a monogenic autoimmune disease providing new clues to self-tolerance. Immunol Today 1998;19; 384-386.

[lxiv] Shimaka N, Nusspaumer G, Holländer GA. Clearing the AIRE: on the pathophysiological basis of the autoimmune polyendocrinopathy syndrome type-1. Endocrinol Metab Clin North Am. 2009; 38: 273-88, vii.

[lxv] Von Schnurbein J, Lahr G, Posovszky C, Debatin KM, Wabitsch M. Novel homozygous AIRE mutation in a German patient with severe APECED. J Pediatr Endocrinol Metab. 2008; 21: 1003-9.

[lxvi] Lawrence T, Puel A, Reichenbach J, et al. Autosomal-dominant primary immunodeficiencies. Curr Opin Hematol 2005;12; 22-30.

[lxvii] Atkinson TP, Schaffer B, Grimbacher B, et al. An immune defect causing dominant mucocutaneous candidiasis and thyroid disease maps to chromosome 2p in a single family. Am J Hum Genet 2002;69; 791-803.

[lxviii] Nahum A, Bates A, Sharfe N, Roifman CM. Association of the lymphoid protein tyrosine phosphatase, R620W variant, with chronic mucocutaneous candidiasis. J Allergy Clin Immunol. 2008; 12: 1220-2.

[lxix] Klein RS, Harris CA, Small CR, Moll B, Lesser M, Friedland GH. Oral candidiasis in high-risk patients as the initial manifestation of the acquired immune deficiency syndrome. N Eng J Med. 1984; 311: 354-8.

[lxx] Zlogotora J, Shapiro MS. Polyglandular autoimmune syndrome type I among Jews. J Med Genet. 1992; 29: 824-6.

[lxxi] Rosatelli MC, Meloni A, Meloni A, Devoto M, Cao A, Scott HS, Peterson P, Heino M, Krohn KJ, Nagamine K, Kudoh J, Shimizu N, Antonarakis SE. A common mutation in Sardinian autoimmune polyendocrinopathy-candidiasis-ectodermal dystrophy patients. Hum Genet. 1998; 103: 428-34.

[lxxii] Ahonen P, Myllärniemi S, Sipilä I, Perheentupa J. Clinical variation of autoimmune polyendocrinopathy-candidiasis-ectodermal dystrophy (APECED) in a series of 68 patients. N Eng J Med. 1990; 322: 1829-36.

[lxxiii] Björses P, Aaltonen J, Vikman A, Perheentupa J, Ben-Zion G, Chiumello G, Dahl N, Heideman P, Hoorweg-Nijman JJ, Mathivon L, Mullis PE, Pohl M, Ritzen M, Romeo G, Shapiro MS, Smith CS, Solyom J, Zlotogora J, Peltonen L. Genetic homogeneity of autoimmune polyglandular disease type I. Am J Hum Genet. 1996; 59: 879-86.

[lxxiv] Wolff AS, Erichsen MM, Meager A, Magitta NF, Myhre AG, Bollerslev J, Fougner KJ, Lima K, Knappskog PM, Husebye ES. Autoimmune polyendocrinopathy syndrome type 1 in Norway: phenotypic variation, autoantibodies, and novel mutations in the autoimmune regulator gene. J Clin Endocrinol Metab. 2007; 92: 595-603.

[lxxv] Lilic D, Gravenor I. Immunology of chronic mucocutaneous candidiasis. J Clin Pathol 2001;54; 81-83.

[lxxvi] Walker SM, Urbaniak SJ. A serum-dependent defect of neutrophil function in chronic mucocutaneous candidiasis. J Clin Pathol 1980;33; 370-372.

[lxxvii] Eyerich K, Rombold S, Foerster S, Behrendt H, Hofmann H, Ring J, et al (2007). Altered, but not diminished T cell response in chronic mucocutaneous candidiasis patients. *Arch Derm Res*, 299:475-81.

[lxxviii] Challacombe SJ. Immunologic aspects of oral candidiasis. Oral Surg Oral Med Oral Pathol 1994;78; 202-10.

[lxxix] Yamazaki M, Yasui K, Kawai H, et al. A monocyte disorder in siblings with chronic candidiasis. A combined abnormality of monocyte mobility and phagocytosis-killing ability. Am J Dis Child 1984;138; 192-6.

[lxxx] Ashman RB, Papadimitriou JM. Production and function of cytokines in natural and acquired immunity to Candida albicans infection. Microbiol Rev 1995; 59; 646-72.

[lxxxi] Palma-Carlos AG, Palma-Carlos ML, da Silva SL. Natural killer (NK) cells in mucocutaneous candidiasis. Allerg Immunol (Paris) 2002;34; 208-12.

[lxxxii] De Moraes-Vasconcelos D, Orii NM, Romano CC, et al. Characterization of the cellular immune function of patients with chronic mucocutaneous candidiasis. Clin Exp Immunol

2001;123; 247-253.

lxxxiii Lilic D, Calvert JE, Cant AJ, et al. Chronic mucocutaneous candidiasis. II. Class and subclass of specific antibody responses in vivo and in vitro. Clin Exp Immunol 1996;105; 213-219.

lxxxiv Bentur L, Nesbet-Brown E, Levinson H, Roifman CM. Lung disease associated with IgG subclass deficiency in chronic mucocutaneous candidiasis. J Pediatr 1991;118; 82-6.

lxxxv IUIS scientific group. Primary immunodeficiency diseases. Clin Exp Immunol 1999;118(suppl 1); 17.

lxxxvi De Moraes-Vasconcelos D, Orii NM, Romano CC, et al. Characterization of the cellular immune function of patients with chronic mucocutaneous candidiasis. Clin Exp Immunol 2001;123; 247-253.

lxxxvii Mencacci A, Perruccio K, Bacci A, Cenci E, Benedetti R, Martelli MF, et al (2001). Defective antifungal t-helper 1 (TH1) immunity in a murine model of allogeneic T-cell-depleted bone marrow transplantation and its restoration by treatment with TH2 cytokine antagonists. *Blood* 97: 1483-90.

lxxxviii Tavares D, Ferreira P, Arala-Chaves M (2000). Increased resistance to systemic candidiasis in athymic or Interleukin-10-depleted mice. *J Infect Dis* 182: 266-73.

lxxxix Huang W, Na L, Fidel PL, Schwarzenberger P (2004). Requirement of Interleukin-17A for systemic anti-Candida albicans host defense in mice. J Infect Dis 190: 624-31.

xc Acosta-Rodriguez EV, Rivino L, Geginat J, Jarrossay D, Gattorno M, Lanzavecchia A, et al (2007). Surface phenotype and antigenic specificity of human interleukin 17-producing T helper memory cells. *Nat Immunol* 8: 639-46.

xci Conti HR, Shen F, Nayyar N, Stocum E, Sun JN, Lindemann MJ, Ho AW, Hai JH, Yu JJ, Jung JW, Filler SG, Masso-Welch P, Edgerton M, Gaffen SL. Th17 cells and IL-17 receptor signaling are essential for mucosal host defense against oral candidiasis. J Exp Med. 2009; 206: 299-311.

xcii Lilic D, Gravenor I, Robson N, et al. Deregulated production of protective cytokines in response to Candida albicans infection in patients with chronic mucocutaneous candidiasis. Infect Immun 2003;71; 5690-5699.

xciii Lilic D, Cant AJ, Abinun M, et al. Chronic mucocutaneous candidiasis. I. Altered antigen-stimulated IL-2, IL-4, IL-6 and interferon-gamma (IFN-□) production. Clin Exp Immunol 1996;105; 205-212.

xciv Van der Graaf CAA, Netea MG, Drenth JPH, et al. Candida-specific interferon-□ deficiency and Toll-like receptor polymorphisms in patients with chronic mucocutaneous candidiasis. Neth J Med 2003;61; 365-369.

[xcv] Kobrynski LJ, Tanimune L, Kilpatrick L, et al. Production of T-helper cell subsets and cytokines by lymphocytes from patients with chronic mucocutaneous candidiasis. Clin Diagn Lab Immunol 1996;3; 740-745.

[xcvi] Ryan KR, Hong M, Arkwright PD, Gennery AR, Costigan C, Dominguez M, Denning D, McConnell V, Cant AJ, Abinun M, Spickett GP, Lilic D. Impaired dendritic cell maturation and cytokine production in patients with chronic mucocutaneous candidiasis with or without APECED. Clin Exp Immunol. 2008; 154: 406-14.

[xcvii] Hong M, Ryan KR, Arkwright PD, Gennery AR, Costigan C, Dominguez M, Denning DW, McConnell V, Cant AJ, Abinun M, Spickett GP, Swan DC, Gillespie CS, Young DA, Lilic D. Clin Exp Immunol. 2009; 156: 40-51.

[xcviii] Lingelbach A, Seidl HP, Frimberger E, Traidl-Hoffmann C, Ring J, Hofmann H. Chronic mucocutaneous candidosis with severe esophageal stricture. Mycoses. 2003; 46 Suppl 1; 15-8.

[xcix] McGurk M, Holmes M. Chronic muco-cutaneous candidiasis and oral neoplasia. J Laryngol Otol. 1988; 102: 643-5.

[c] Firth NA, O'Grady JF, Reade PC. Oral squamous cell carcinoma in a young person with candidosis endocrinopathy syndrome: a case report. Int J Oral Maxillofac Surg. 1997; 26: 42-4.

[ci] Rosa DD, Pasqualotto AC, Denning DW. Chronic mucocutaneous candidiasis and oesophageal cancer. Med Mycol. 2008; 46: 85-91.

[cii] Malfertheiner P, Peitz U. The interplay between Helicobacter pylori, gastro-oesophageal reflux disease, and intestinal metaplasia. Gut 2005;54 Suppl1: 13-20.

[ciii] Eyerich K, Traidl-Hoffmann C, Albert A, Kerzl R, Rombold S, Darsow U, Everlein B, Jakob T, Ring J, Hein R. Lipomatous metaplasia after severe and chronic cutaneous inflammation. Dermatology. 2008; 217: 52-5.

[civ] Valdimarsson H, Moss PD, Holt PJ, H Obbs JR. Treatment of chronic mucocutaneous candidiasis with leukocytes from HL-A compatible sibling. Lancet.

[cv] Levy RL, Bach ML, Huang S, Bach FH, Hong R, Ammann AJ, Bortin M, Kay HE. Thymic transplantation in a case of chronic mucocutaneous candidiasis. Lancet. 1971; 2: 898-900.

[cvi] Chapman SW, Sullivan DC, Cleary JD. In search of the holy grail of antifungal therapy. Trans Am Clin Climatol Assoc. 2008; 119: 197-215.

[cvii] Rautemaa R et al. Activity of amphotericin b, anidulafungin, caspofungin, micafungin, and voriconazole against Candida albicans with decreased susceptibility to fluconazole from APECED patients on long-term azole treatment of chronic mucocoutaneous candidiasis. Diagn Mircrobial Infect Dis. 2008; 62: 182-5.

[cviii] Sabatelli F, Patel R, Mann PA, Mednrick CA, Norris CC, Hare R, Loebenberg D, Black TA, McNicholas PM. In vitro activities of posaconazole, fluconazole, itraconazole, voriconazole, and amphotericin B against a large collection of clinically important molds and yeasts. Antimircob Agents Chemother. 2006; 50: 2009-15.

[cix] Cappelletty D, Eiselstein-McKitrick K. The echinocandins. Pharmacotherapy. 2007; 27: 369-88.

[cx] McCormack PL, Perry CM. Caspofungin: a review of its use in the treatment of fungal infections. Drugs. 2005; 65: 2049-68.

[cxi] Cross SA, Scott LJ. Micafungin: a review of its use in adults for the treatment of invasive and oesophageal candidiasis, and as prophylaxis against Candida infections. Drugs. 2008; 68: 2225-55.

[cxii] Moen MD, Lysen-Williamson KA, Scott LJ. Liposomal amphotericin B: a review of its use as empirical therapy in febrile neutropenia and in the treatment of invasive fungal infections. Drugs. 2009; 69: 361-92.

[cxiii] Leung DY, Bonguniewicz M, Howell MD, Nomura I, Hamid QA. New insights into atopic dermatitis. J Clin Invest 2004;113:651-7.

[cxiv] Leung AK, Hon KL, Robson WL. Atopic dermatitis. Adv Pediatr 2007;54:241-73.

[cxv] Bach JF. The effect of infections on susceptibility to autoimmune and allergic diseases. N Engl J Med 2002;347:911-20.

[cxvi] Braback L, Hjern A, Rasmussen F. Trends in asthma, allergic rhinitis and eczema among swedish conscripts from farming and non-farming enviroments. A nationwide study over three decades. Clin Exp Allergy 2004;34:38-43.

[cxvii] Leung DY, Bieber T. Atopic dermatitis. Lancet 2003;361:151-160.

[cxviii] Palmer CN, Irvine AD, Terron-Kwiatkowski A, Zhao Y, Liao H, Lee SP, et al. Common loss-of-function variants of the epidermal barrier protein filaggrin are a major predisposing factor for atopic dermatitis. Nat Genet 2006;38:441-6.

[cxix] Weidinger S, O´Sullivan M, Illig T, Baurecht H, Depner M, Rodriguez E, et al. Filaggrin mutations, atopic eczema, hay fever, and asthma in children. J Allergy Clin Immunol 2008;121:1203-9.

[cxx] Ring J, Darsow U, Gfesser M, Vieluf D. The ´atopy patch test´ in evaluating the role of aeroallergens in atopic eczema. Int Arch Allergy Immunol 1997;113:379-83.

[cxxi] Grewe M, Walther S, Gyufko K, Czech W, Schopf E, Krutmann J. Analysis of the cytokine pattern expressed in situ in inhalant allergen patch test reactions of atopic dermatitis patients. J Invest Dermatol 1995;105:407-10.

[cxxii] Eyerich K, Huss-Marp J, Darsow U, Wollenberg A, Foerster S, Ring J, et al. Pollen grains induce a rapid and biphasic eczematous immune response in atopic eczema patients. Int Arch Allergy Immunol 2008;145:213-22.

[cxxiii] Ong PY, Ohtake T, Brandt C, Strickland I, Boguniewicz M, Ganz T, et al. Endogenous antimicrobial peptides and skin infections in atopic dermatitis. N Eng J Med 2002;347:1151-60.

[cxxiv] Mempel M, Lina G, Hojka M, Schnopp C, Seidl HP, Schafer T, et al. High prevalence of superantigens associated with the egc locus in Staphylococcus aureus isolates from patients with atopic eczema. Eur J Clin Microbiol Infect Dis 2003;22:306-9.

[cxxv] Bunikowski R, Mielke ME, Skarabis H, Worm M, Anagnostopoulos I, Kolde G, et al. Evidence for a disease-promoting effect of Staphylococcus aureus-derived exotoxins in atopic dermatitis. J Allergy Clin Immunol 2000;105:814-9.

[cxxvi] Choi Y, Kotzin B, Herron L, Callahan J, Marrack P, Kappler J. Interaction of Staphylococcus aureus toxin "superantigens" with human T cells. Proc Natl Acad Sci USA 1989;86:8941-5.

[cxxvii] Langer K, Breuer K, Kapp A, Werfel T. Staphylococcus aureus-derived enterotoxins enhance house dust mite-induced patch test reactions in atopic dermatitis. Exp Dermatol 2007;16:124-129.

[cxxviii] 41st World Medical Assembly (1997). Declaration of Helsinki: recommendations guiding physicians in biomedical reasearch involving human subjects. *JAMA* 277: 925-926.

[cxxix] Hanifin JM: Basic and clinical aspects of atopic dermatitis. Ann Allergy 1984; 52:386-395.

[cxxx] Darsow U, Ring J: Airborne and dietary allergens in atopic eczema: a comprehensive review of diagnostic tests. Clin Exp Dermatol 2000; 25:544-551.

[cxxxi] LeibundGut-Landmann S, Groß O, Robinson MJ, Osorio F, Slack EO, Tsoni SV, et al (2007). Syk- and CARD9-dependent coupling of innate immunity to the induction of T helper cells that produce interleukin 17. *Nat Immunol* 8: 630-38.

[cxxxii] Xie MH, Aggarwal S, Ho WH, Foster J, Zhang Z, Stinson J, et al (2000) Interleukin (IL)-22, a novel human cytokine that signals through the interferon receptor-related proteins CRF2-4 and IL-22R. *J Biol Chem* 275:31335-9.

[cxxxiii] Kreymborg K, Etzensperger R, Dumoutier L, Haak S, Rebollo A, Buch T, et al (2007). IL-22 is expressed by Th17 cells in an IL-23-dependent fashion, but not required for the development of autoimmune encephalomyelitis. *J Immunol* 179: 8098-104

[cxxxiv] Veldhoen M, Hocking RJ, Atkins CJ, Locksley RM, Stockinger B (2006). TGF☐ in the context of an inflammatory cytokine milieu supports de novo differentiation of IL-17-

producing T cells. *Immunity* 24; 179-189.

[cxxxv] Evans HG, Suddason T, Jackson I, Taams LS, Lord GM (2007). Optimal induction of T helper 17 cells in humans requires T cell receptor ligation in the context of Toll-like receptor-activated monocytes. *Proc Natl Acad Sci USA* 104: 17034-9.

[cxxxvi] Feng Z, Jiang B, Chandra J, Ghannoum M, Nelson S, Weinberg A (2005). Human beta-defensins: differential activity against candidal species and regulation by Candida albicans. *J Dent Res* 84: 445-50.

[cxxxvii] Vylkova S, Nayyar N, Li W, Edgerton M (2007). Human beta-defensins kill Candida albicans in an energy-dependent and salt-sensitive manner without causing membrane disruption. *Antimicrob Agents Chemother* 51: 154-61.

[cxxxviii] Howell MD, Boguniewicz M, Pastore S, Novak N, Bieber T, Girolomoni G, et al. Mechanism of HBD-3 deficiency in atopic dermatitis. Clin Immunol 2006;121:332-38.

[cxxxix] Albanesi C, Fairchild HR, Madonna S, Scarponi C, De Pità O, Leung DY, Howell MD. IL-4 and IL-13 negatively regulate TNF-alpha- and IFN-gamma-induced beta-defensin expression through STAT-6, suppressor of cytokine signaling (SOCS)-1, and SOCS-3. J Immunol 2007;179:984-92.

[cxl] Minegishi Y, Saito M, Nagasawa M, Takada H, Hara T, Tsuchiya S, Agematsu K, Yamada M, Kawamura N, Ariga T, Tsuge I, Karasuyama H. Molecular explanation for the correlation between systemic Th17 defect and localized bacterial infection in hyper-IgE syndrome. J Exp Med. 2009; 206: 1291-301.

[cxli] Milner JD, Brenchley JM, Laurence A, Freeman AF, Hill BJ, Elias KM, et al. Impaired Th17 cell differentiation in subjects with autosomal dominant hyper-IgE syndrome. Nature 2008;452:733-6.

[cxlii] Toda M, Leung DY, Molet S, Boguniewicz M, Taha R, Christodoulopoulos P, Polarized in vivo expression of IL-11 and IL-17 between acute and chronic skin lesions. J Allergy Clin Immunol 2003;111:875-81.

[cxliii] Annunziato F, Cosmi L, Santarlasci V, Maggi L, Liotta F, Mazzinghi B, et al. Phenotypic and functional features of human Th17 cells. J Exp Med 2007;204:1849-61.

[cxliv] Chen Y, Langrish CL, McKenzie B, Joyce-Shaikh B, Stumhofer JS, McClanahan T, et al. Anti-IL-23 therapy inhibits multiple inflammatory pathways and ameliorates autoimmune encephalomyelitis. J Clin Invest 2006;116:1317-26.

[cxlv] Howell MD, Boguniewicz M, Pastore S, Novak N, Bieber T, Girolomoni G, et al. Mechanism of HBD-3 deficiency in atopic dermatitis. Clin Immunol 2006;121:332-38.

[cxlvi] Albanesi C, Fairchild HR, Madonna S, Scarponi C, De Pità O, Leung DY, Howell MD. IL-4 and IL-13 negatively regulate TNF-alpha- and IFN-gamma-induced beta-defensin

expression through STAT-6, suppressor of cytokine signaling (SOCS)-1, and SOCS-3. J Immunol 2007;179:984-92

[cxlvii] Grewe M, Walther S, Gyufko K, Czech W, Schopf E, Krutmann J. Analysis of the cytokine pattern expressed in situ in inhalant allergen patch test reactions of atopic dermatitis patients. J Invest Dermatol 1995;105:407-10.

[cxlviii] Howell MD, Kim BE, Gao P, Grant AV, Boguniewicz M, DeBenedetto A, Schneider L, Beck LA, Banres KC, Leung DY. Cytokine modulation of atopic dermatitis filaggrin skin epxression. J Allergy Clin Immunol. 2009; 124(3 suppl 2): R7-R12.

[cxlix] Oyoshi MK, Murphy GF, Geha RS. Filaggrin-deficient mice exhibit TH17-dominated skin inflammation and permissiveness to epicutaneous sensitization with protein antigen. J Allergy Clin Immunol. 2009; 124: 494-5.

[cl] Traidl C, Sebastiani S, Albanesi C, Merk HF, Puddu P, Girolomoni G, et al. Disparate cytotoxic activity of nickel-specific CD8+ and CD4+ T cell subsets against keratinocytes. J Immunol 2000;165:3058-3064.

[cli] Trautmann A, Altznauer F, Akdis M, Simon HU, Disch R, Bröcker EB, et al. The differential fate of cadherins during T-cell-induced keratinocyte apoptosis leads to spongiosis in eczematous dermatitis. J Invest Dermatol 2001;117:927-34.


## 8    Acknowledgement


This book is a reprint of the Ph.D. thesis that was granted by the Technical University Munich in 2010. Scientific research is a rapidly evolving and complex field. Consequently, gained knowledge and insights into clinical pathomechanisms results from the collaboration of many people working closely together.

In that context I want to express my gratitude towards my scientific mentors, PD Claudia Traidl-Hoffmann and Prof. Andrea Cavani first. I am grateful to Prof. Heidrun Behrendt and Prof. Johannes Ring who always supported me on my way. These four may stand for the numerous people that helped and advised me at the ZAUM – center for allergy and environment and the clinic for dermatology and allergology Biederstein as well as the Istituto Dermopatico Dell'Immacolata. One person, however, I want to thank at the prominent last position: my source of peace and power, my reasonable mirror and inspiring partner. Our close interaction has produced the best one can think of.

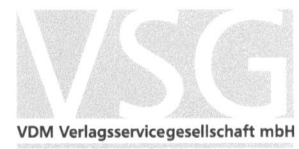

Die VDM Verlagsservicegesellschaft sucht für wissenschaftliche Verlage abgeschlossene und herausragende

## Dissertationen, Habilitationen, Diplomarbeiten, Master Theses, Magisterarbeiten usw.

für die kostenlose Publikation als Fachbuch.

Sie verfügen über eine Arbeit, die hohen inhaltlichen und formalen Ansprüchen genügt, und haben Interesse an einer honorarvergüteten Publikation?

Dann senden Sie bitte erste Informationen über sich und Ihre Arbeit per Email an *info@vdm-vsg.de*.

**Sie erhalten kurzfristig unser Feedback!**

VDM Verlagsservicegesellschaft mbH
Dudweiler Landstr. 99
D - 66123 Saarbrücken

Telefon +49 681 3720 174
Fax +49 681 3720 1749

**www.vdm-vsg.de**

Die VDM Verlagsservicegesellschaft mbH vertritt

 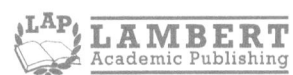 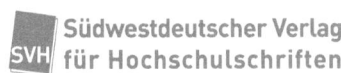

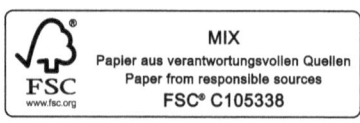

Printed by Books on Demand GmbH, Norderstedt / Germany